UNDERSTAND

ECG

A GUIDE FOR NURSES

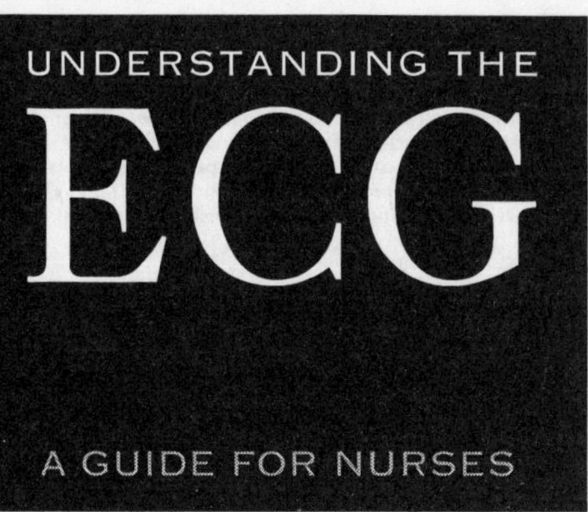

ERICA NASH &
VIOLETTA NAHAS

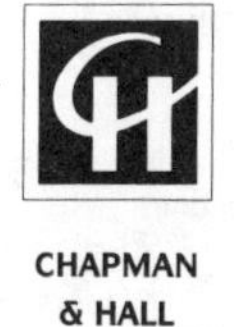

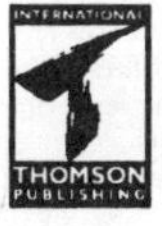

An International Thomson Publishing Company

Melbourne • Bonn • Boston • London • Madrid • Mexico City • New York • Paris • Singapore
Tokyo • Toronto • Albany NY • Belmont CA • Cincinnati OH • Detroit MI

First published in Australia in 1996 by
Thomas Nelson Australia
102 Dodds Street
South Melbourne 3205

Simultaneously published in the United Kingdom for distribution outside
Australia, New Zealand and North America by
Chapman & Hall
2–6 Boundary Row
London SE1 8HN

ISBN 0-412-75310-3

I Ⓣ P Thomas Nelson Australia and Chapman & Hall are imprints of International
Thomson Publishing company

10 9 8 7 6 5 4 3 2 1
99 98 97 96

National Library of Australia
Cataloguing-in-Publication data

Nash, Erica
Understanding the ECG: a guide for nurses.
Includes index.
ISBN 0 17 008927 4.
1. Electrocardiography. 2. Heart - Diseases - Nursing. 3. Electrocardiography - Problems, exercises, etc. 4. Heart - Diseases - Nursing Problems, exercises, etc. I. Nahas, Violetta. II. Title. III. Title: Understanding electrocardiography.
616.1207547

A catalogue record for this book is
available from the British Library

Cover designed by Deborah Gilkes
Text designed by Deborah Gilkes
Illustrated by Alan Laver, Shelley Communications
Typeset by J & M Typesetters
Printed in Australia by Australian Print Group

Nelson Australia Pty Limited ACN 004 603 454 (incorporated in Victoria) trading as
Thomas Nelson Australia.

The I Ⓣ P trademark is used under licence.

Within the publishing process Thomas Nelson Australia uses resources, technology and
suppliers that are as environmentally friendly as possible.

CONTENTS

Preface		vii
Acknowledgements		ix
Chapter 1	**Overview of cardiac anatomy and physiology**	1
	Objectives	1
	Key words	1
	Cardiac anatomy	2
	Cardiac physiology	6
	The heart's conduction system	9
	Cardiac haemodynamics	10
	References	12
Chapter 2	**Electrocardiography**	14
	Objectives	14
	Key words	14
	Electrocardiography	15
	Electrocardiograph paper	15
	The electrocardiogram	17
	Leads and their positions	18
	Wave deflections	20
	The heart's electrical axis	28
	Interpreting the cardiac rhythm	29
	References	39
Chapter 3	**Techniques used to record the cardiac rhythm**	41
	Objectives	41
	Key words	41
	Monitoring the heart's electrical pattern	42
	Lead placement	46
	Procedure for attaching a patient to a cardiac monitor	48
	Exercise electrocardiography	49
	Electrophysiological studies	52
	References	56
Chapter 4	**Common arrhythmias**	57
	Objectives	57
	Key words	57
	Critical incident	58
	Sinus rhythm	58
	Arrhythmias of the sinoatrial node	60

	Arrhythmias of the atria	66
	Junctional arrhythmias	71
	Ventricular arrhythmias	76
	Atrioventricular blocks (conduction disorders)	84
	Bundle branch blocks	90
	Exercises — cardiac rhythm interpretation	95
	References	96
Chapter 5	**Nursing management of patients with arrhythmias**	98
	Objectives	98
	Key words	98
	Critical incident	99
	Assessment	99
	Common nursing diagnosis	109
	Electrical therapy for arrhythmias	115
	References	129
Chapter 6	**Interpreting a myocardial infarction from a 12 lead ECG**	132
	Objectives	132
	Key words	132
	Case study	133
	What is a myocardial infarction?	133
	How is a myocardial infarction diagnosed?	135
	Electrocardiographic changes following an acute myocardial infarction	137
	Interpretation of a myocardial infarction from a 12 lead ECG	145
	References	147
Chapter 7	**Exercises in cardiac rhythm and 12 lead ECG interpretation**	149
	Part A — cardiac rhythm interpretation	149
	Part B — 12 lead ECG interpretation	165
Appendix 1	**Answers to exercises (Chapter 4)**	172
Appendix 2	**Answers to exercises (Chapter 7)**	174
	Part A — cardiac rhythm interpretation	174
	Part B — 12 lead ECG interpretation	187
Glossary		193
Index		203

PREFACE

Over the past 30 years advances in medical technology have brought about changes in the way patients are managed. Ten years ago patients may have been admitted to hospital for up to a week to undergo a battery of investigations — today, many minor procedures can be performed safely in the practitioner's room with the client presenting as a 'day only' patient. Likewise, some acutely ill patients can now be cared for outside of specialist units due to developments in the use of cardiac monitoring.

To keep abreast of these changes and to ensure that an optimum level of care is delivered to the patient, nurses have had to expand their knowledge base and develop appropriate skills in nursing management. Learning to interpret cardiac rhythms and 12 lead electrocardiograms (ECGs) should no longer be seen as the domain of clinical nurse specialists working in areas such as intensive care or the emergency department. This skill should be developed by every nurse involved with patient assessment.

PURPOSE

Understanding the ECG — A Guide for Nurses was conceived when we were teaching the critical care component of the Diploma (now Degree) of Applied Science for undergraduate nursing students. While teaching basic electrocardiography we discovered that the recommended texts did not meet students' needs. The students also felt that if they had a text which met the requirements of the course, it would be helpful for immediate use and for when they had graduated and were caring for the community.

To address this situation we developed a book, *Electrocardiography for Nursing Students — A Study Manual*, to support lecture and tutorial notes, and to be used as an adjunct to more detailed literature on the subject. The feedback we received from undergraduate and postgraduate students was very encouraging, and so we decided to have the manual published with some alterations to its content and format.

Understanding the ECG — A Guide for Nurses is ideal for use by students enrolled in multidiscipline courses, such as undergraduate and postgraduate nursing students, medical students, students enrolled in ECG technician courses conducted by colleges of TAFE; staff employed in health fund centres who are involved with heart programs; and allied health professional groups, such as the ambulance service. *Understanding the ECG — A Guide for Nurses* is also appropriate for use by interested members of the community.

STRUCTURE

Understanding the ECG — A Guide for Nurses consists of seven chapters. Chapter 1 gives a basic overview of cardiac anatomy and physiology. Chapter 2 discusses the basic principles of electrocardiography and then applies these principles to the practice of interpreting cardiac rhythms. Chapter 3 discusses the methods used to record cardiac rhythms and the responsibilities of staff caring for patients being monitored. Chapter 4 describes the basic cardiac arrhythmias, their main characteristics, and the current nursing and medical management required. Beside the electrocardiograph of each arrhythmia is an example of a normal sinus rhythm electrocardiograph for you to compare. You have the opportunity to practise cardiac rhythm interpretation by attempting the exercises included at the end of Chapter 4. Answers are provided in Appendix 1. Chapter 5 discusses in more detail the nursing management required for patients presenting with arrhythmias and describes the main electrical interventions used, including cardioversion, emergency defibrillation and cardiac pacing. We have adopted a general approach to nursing management because we recognise that each health facility has its own protocol on patient care.

Chapter 6 discusses myocardial infarctions and how to interpret these from a 12 lead ECG. Additional practice in interpreting cardiac rhythms can be gained from attempting the exercises in Chapter 7 and checking the answers in Appendix 2.

A Glossary which defines terms discussed in the text is located at the back of the book.

ACKNOWLEDGEMENTS

We gratefully acknowledge the support and assistance of our families, friends and colleagues in making this book possible. In particular, we appreciate the assistance of Jane Cooper, Clinical Nurse Specialist, who generously gave her personal time to discuss current nursing management and check our ECG interpretations; to Pat Johnson, lecturer and a former ICU course coordinator, for supplying some of the 12 lead ECGs and giving us permission to expand her myocardial infarction table which has been included in Chapter 6; and to Troy Burke, Clinical/Technical Manager of Telectronics (Sydney), for assisting us with information regarding the implantable cardioverter/defibrillator.

We would like to thank all the reviewers for painstakingly reading our manuscript and offering many worthwhile suggestions for us to consider while compiling the text. We would especially like to thank Hannelore Best, Senior Lecturer, Faculty of Nursing, University of Ballarat, for reading our final draft of the manuscript and for her thoughtful insights.

A special thankyou is extended to the staff of Thomas Nelson Australia, especially Peter Demery, Academic Representative, who saw our study manual and encouraged us to try for publication; to Lee Walker, Editor; and to Julie McNab, Senior Acquisitions Editor, for her encouragement and commitment to excellence.

Finally, we wish to express our gratitude to our husbands, Jim and Shaker, for their love and support, and to our children, Andrew, Ali, Alia, Aisha and Amira, for their patience while we were busy writing this book.

Erica Nash, Lecturer
Department of Nursing Practice
School of Nursing and Human Movement
Australian Catholic University, Sydney

Violetta Nahas, Lecturer
Department of Community Nursing and Mental Health
School of Nursing
Cumberland College of Health Sciences, University of Sydney

{1}

OVERVIEW OF CARDIAC ANATOMY AND PHYSIOLOGY

OBJECTIVES

After working through this chapter you should be able to:

- describe the anatomical structure of the heart
- describe the blood flow through the heart
- describe the normal cardiac conduction system
- discuss cardiac physiology and relate these processes to the heart's conduction system
- discuss the relationship between the mechanical events and the electrical events of the cardiac cycle

KEY WORDS

afterload
aorta
aortic valve
atrium
automaticity
cardiac cycle
cardiac output
chordae tendineae
compliance
conductivity
contractility
coronary artery
diastole
endocardium
epicardium
excitability
mitral valve
myocardium
papillary muscles
pericardium
preload
pulmonary artery
pulmonary valve
refractoriness
sinoatrial node
stroke volume
systole
tricuspid valve
ventricle

CARDIAC ANATOMY

The heart is a hollow, cone-shaped muscular organ situated in the space between the lungs which is called the *mediastinum.* It weighs approximately 300 g and is about the size of the owner's clenched fist. The heart consists of three layers of tissue. These are the *endocardium*, *myocardium* and *epicardium.*

Endocardium consists of endothelial tissue that lines the interior surface of the heart and the cardiac valves.

Myocardium is the middle layer of heart tissue and consists of bundles of striated muscle fibres. There are three main types of myocardial muscles: the atrial and ventricular muscles and the specialised muscle fibres. Myocardial muscles are involved in the work of excitation and conduction.

Epicardium covers the external surface of the heart and consists of a layer of mesothelial cells. This tissue extends a short way along the aorta and the pulmonary artery and amalgamates with the tunica adventitia of these vessels before doubling back upon itself to become the parietal pericardium. It is this continuous membrane which forms the pericardial sac containing approximately 20 mL of clear serous fluid. This fluid lubricates the parietal and visceral pericardia as they slide across each other during the systole phase.

The pericardium also helps to hold the heart in its position in the chest cavity and prevents the spread of infection and neoplastic disease to the heart from other areas of the body.

The pericardium consists of two layers of tissue: the inner layer, called the serous parietal; and the outer layer, which is tough and fibrous and called the pericardial membrane. The pericardial membrane can also be found attached to the ligaments of the sternum and the diaphragm (Underhill et al 1989, p 17).

The heart's main functions are: firstly, to pump blood, oxygen and nutrients through the body via a system of arteries, arterioles and capillaries; and secondly, to collect and transport deoxygenated blood via veins and venules to the lungs where carbon dioxide is extracted from it and the oxygen replenished.

CHAMBERS

The heart has four chambers. The upper chambers are called the *atria* (*sing* atrium) and the lower chambers are called *ventricles.* There is a paired atrium and ventricle on each side of the heart. These are separated from one another by a muscular wall called the *septum.* The atria act as reservoirs or collecting chambers for blood before it passes through the valves into the ventricles. The right atrium receives deoxygenated blood from the body via the superior and inferior vena cava. From here, blood flows into the right ventricle through the tricuspid valve. From the right ventricle, the blood is pumped through the pulmonary valve into the pulmonary artery and then to the lungs where carbon dioxide is exchanged for oxygen. The oxygenated blood enters the left atrium via the four pulmonary veins. (The pulmonary veins are the only veins in the body that transport oxygenated blood.) The blood passes through the mitral valve into the left ventricle and is ejected through the aortic valve into the aorta. The aorta distributes the blood to the body via a system of arterioles and capillaries (see Figure 1.1).

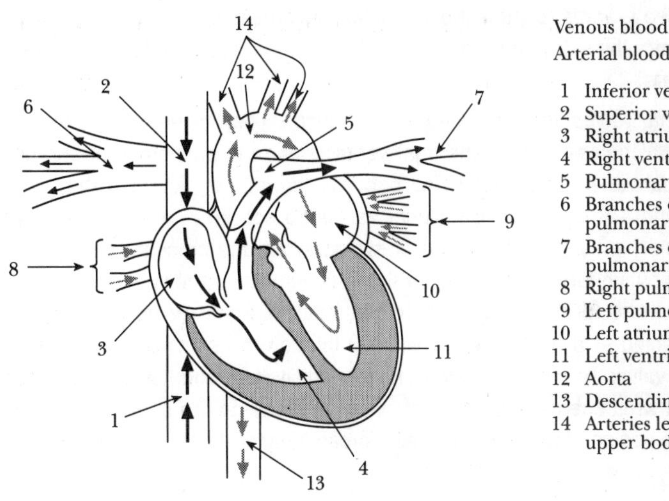

FIGURE 1.1 *Blood flow through the heart*

The walls of the left ventricle are at least two and a half times thicker than the walls of the right ventricle. This is because the left ventricle has to eject blood into the body where the systematic circulation offers a greater vascular resistance than when the right ventricle ejects blood into the lung fields.

VALVES

The cardiac valves are located between the atria and the ventricles, and the ventricles and their corresponding artery. Their function is to ensure that blood flows in one direction only (see Figure 1.2). Valves are composed of thin leaves of fibrous tissue and open and close in response to pressure changes between the atria and the ventricles, the aorta and the pulmonary artery. There are two types of cardiac valves:

(i) *Atrioventricular valves* (AV valves) separate the atria from the ventricles. The *tricuspid valve*, so-called because it has three cusps, separates the right atrium from the right ventricle. Between the left atrium and the left ventricle is the *mitral valve*. It has two cusps and is referred to as the *bicuspid valve*. To maintain unidirectional blood flow between the atria and the ventricles, the AV valves are supported by muscle bundles called *papillary muscles* which are embedded in the walls of the ventricles. Attached to the papillary muscles are the *chordae tendineae* which are composed of fibrous bands and extend to the edges of the valve cusps (see Figure 1.2). During systole (contraction), the papillary muscles contract causing the chordae tendineae to become taut. In turn, the valve's cusps are pulled inwards towards the ventricles, preventing the cusps from bulging back into the atria and allowing blood to be regurgitated into these chambers.

(ii) *Semilunar valves* are composed of three cusps. They include the *pulmonary valve,* which lies between the right ventricle and the pulmonary artery, and the *aortic valve,* which is located between the left ventricle and the aorta. Unlike the AV valves, the semilunar valves do not have chordae tendineae or papillary muscles. At the end of systole when the pressure in the aorta and the pulmonary artery is higher than the ventricular pressure, the semilunar valves snap shut rather than close gently like the AV valves. Blood is also ejected at a much greater velocity through the semilunar valves than the AV valves because the area through which the blood flows is narrower. Despite what seems to be a lot of 'wear and tear' on the semilunar valves, they are designed to withstand these forces (Guyton 1991, p 103).

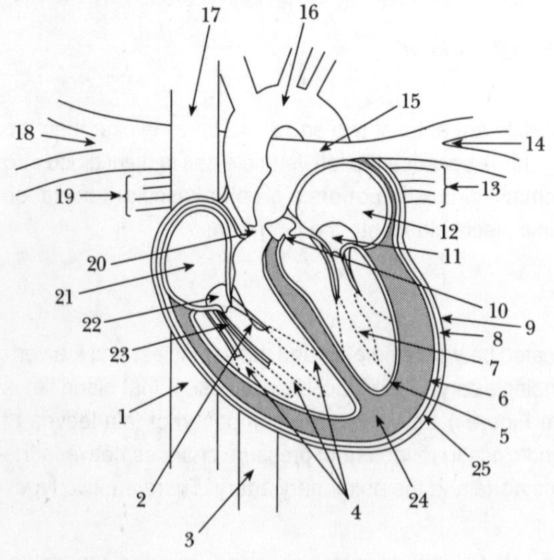

1 Inferior vena cava
2 Right ventricle
3 Descending aorta
4 Papillary muscle
5 Endocardium
6 Epicardium
7 Left ventricle
8 Pericardial space
9 Parietal pericardium
10 Aortic valve
11 Mitral valve
12 Left atrium
13 Left pulmonary veins
14 Branches of left pulmonary artery
15 Pulmonary artery
16 Aorta
17 Superior vena cava
18 Branches of right pulmonary artery
19 Right pulmonary veins
20 Pulmonary valve
21 Right atrium
22 Tricuspid valve
23 Cordae tendineae
24 Myocardium
25 Visceral pericardium

FIGURE 1.2 *Internal structure of the heart*

Source Adapted from Luckman & Sorenson 1987, p 854

To continue moving blood around the body, the heart muscle continually needs replenishment of oxygen and nutrients. *Coronary arteries* are the system of vessels which supply the heart muscle with blood.

The coronary arteries arise in the sinus of Valsalva situated at the base of the aorta near its junction with the left ventricle. The bulk of the left ventricle is supplied by the *left coronary artery* (see Figure 1.3). Branching off from the left coronary artery is the *left anterior descending artery* which passes down the front of the left ventricle. This artery supplies blood to the myocardium of the left ventricle and right ventricle and the interventricular septum. The lateral aspect of the left ventricle and the left atrium are supplied by a branch of the left coronary artery called the *circumflex artery*. The right ventricle receives its blood supply from the *right coronary artery* which runs down the atrioventricular groove between the right atrium and the right ventricle.

The right coronary artery and some of its branches supply blood to the right atrium, the inferior portion of the left ventricle, the posterior section of the septum, and supplies the sinoatrial nodes and the atrioventricular nodes in more than 50% of the human population. Three-quarters of the coronary artery blood flow occurs during diastole (when the heart is relaxed). Venous blood returns from the left ventricle via the *great cardiac vein* which runs parallel to the circumflex artery. This vessel then becomes the *coronary sinus* which empties its contents into the right atrium. Venous blood from the right ventricle is drained via the *anterior cardiac*

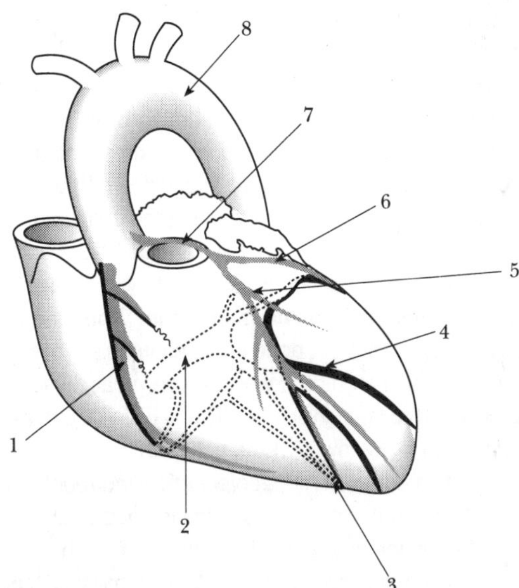

FIGURE 1.3 *Location of the coronary arteries*
Source Adapted from Smeltzer & Bare 1992, p 615

veins directly into the right atrium, bypassing the coronary sinus. A small amount of venous blood drains directly into the ventricles through the *thebesian veins* (Guyton 1991, p 238; Underhill et al 1989, p 24).

NERVE SUPPLY TO THE HEART

Tissues in the heart, such as the coronary artery network or the walls of the ventricles, contain numerous sensory nerve fibres which transmit impulses through the cardiac nerves to the central nervous system. The heart, under the control of the autonomic nervous system, is stimulated by two main groups of nerves.

(i) *Sympathetic nerves* affect the heart by stimulating the sinoatrial node (SA node) to emit impulses at a faster rate, enhancing conduction through the atrioventricular node (AV node), and increasing the heart's force of contraction.

(ii) *Parasympathetic nerves* slow down the rate of impulses leaving the SA node, thus slowing down the rate of conduction through the AV node, and reducing the force of ventricular contraction (Underhill et al 1989, p 25).

CARDIAC PHYSIOLOGY

CHARACTERISTICS OF THE CARDIAC MUSCLE

There are five major electrophysiologic characteristics of the cardiac muscle which maintain the heart's rate and rhythm: *excitability*, *automaticity*, *conductivity*, *refractoriness* and *contractility*.

Excitability is the ability of the cardiac muscle cells to respond to an electrical stimulus. In its resting state the inside of the cell is negative and the outside of the cell is positive, that is, there is a difference in electrical charge across the membrane, which is called the resting membrane potential. The inside of the cell is richer in negative ions, such as proteins and phosphates, and the outside of the cell is richer in positive ions, specifically sodium (Na^+), calcium (Ca^{2+}) and potassium (K^+). There is relatively more sodium outside the cell and more potassium inside, each having its own equilibrium across the membrane. When the cell receives an electrical stimulus (eg when the SA node emits an impulse) of sufficient strength, the membrane will reach a point at which its permeability to the positive ions and hence its potential change significantly. This is called the *threshold* at which an *action potential* occurs (Holloway 1993, p 295–6).

There are two phases of the action potential — *depolarisation* and *repolarisation* — which can be better understood if the ECG complex is used as a guide (see Figure 1.4). At rest, depicted by the isoelectric line on the ECG, the cell's membrane potential is equivalent to approximately –85 to –95 mV (millivolts), but once stimulated the membrane becomes slightly more positive, that is +20 mV. The cause of the altered state of the cell's membrane is attributed to the opening of two types of channels.

(i) *Fast sodium channels* allow for large amounts of sodium ions to diffuse rapidly across the membrane into the cell causing the cell to become positive or depolarised. On the action potential curve this corresponds to Phase 0. Phase 1 — the spike at the tip of Phase 0 — heralds the end of depolarisation and the beginning of early repolarisation when the fast sodium channels are beginning to close.

(ii) *Slow calcium channels* are slower to open than the fast sodium channels. However, they remain open for a longer period of time. Being positively charged, these ions prolong the period of time in which the inside of the cell

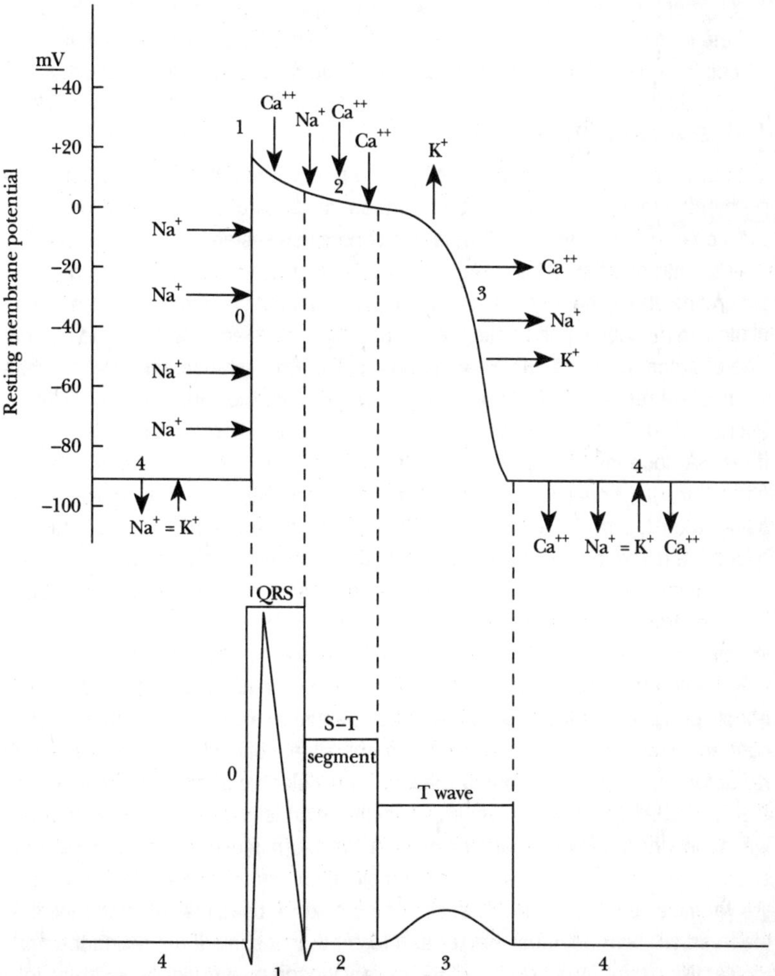

FIGURE 1.4 *The action potential curve in relation to the ECG complex*

remains positive, thereby prolonging the cardiac muscle cells' state of contraction. On the action potential diagram this is represented by the plateau, or Phase 2, and the QRS complex on the ECG. The QRS complex represents transmission of a group of waves created by the passage of the cardiac impulse through the ventricles, the R wave being the most prominent. (It is important to realise that the mechanical events of the heart, such as systole, occur after the electrical events.) Phase 3 represents the closure of the slow channels resulting in a rapid repolarisation. Calcium, sodium and potassium ions efflux, returning the cell to its negative state. Using the ECG complex the space between Phase 2 and Phase 3 corresponds to the ST segment and Phase 3 is the T wave. Now in its resting period — Phase 4 (the isoelectric line on the ECG diagram) — potassium moves back into the cell to equilibrate with the extracellular sodium concentration before the next electrical stimulus arrives (Guyton 1991, pp 101–2; Underhill et al 1989, p 55; Holloway 1992, pp 295–8).

This process, where sodium, calcium and potassium diffuse across the semipermeable membrane, happens throughout all cardiac cells as a positive electrical charge moves through the heart's conduction system.

Automaticity is the ability of the cardiac muscle cells to reach a threshold potential and be able to generate an action potential without the need for external stimulation. In particular, pacemaker cells (specialised cardiac cells) have the highest rate of automaticity (Dienhart et al 1984, p 15). For instance, the SA node has an inherent rate of 60–100 bpm, the junction around the AV node has an inherent rate of 40–60 bpm and the Purkinje fibres have an inherent rate of 20–40 bpm. If the SA node failed to emit an impulse because of trauma or disease, the AV node or the junctional tissue surrounding it would be capable of taking over as the pacemaker for the heart's conduction system because it has the next fastest pacemaker. This pattern continues down the conduction pathways.

Conductivity is the ability of the cardiac muscle cells to transmit electrical impulses from the SA node through the AV node, the bundle of His, the right and left bundle branches and to the Purkinje fibres (Dienhart et al 1984, p 15).

Refractoriness is the heart's ability to maintain a steady rhythm by blocking the effects of a stronger than normal electrical stimulus which would initiate a further contraction by the heart. When the heart is in a state of contraction (the *absolute refractory period*) it is unable to react to a new electrical stimulus (Ignativiticus & Bayne 1991, p 2074). However, when the heart is in the final stages of repolarisation (the *relative refractory period*) the heart muscle can respond to a stronger than normal stimulus. For example, if an ectopic site within the walls of the ventricles emits an impulse ahead of the next SA beat, there is a chance that the heart will contract much earlier and faster than it should, restricting the ventricular filling time. Auscultation of the patient's heart beat during an extrasystole (premature ventricular ectopic beat) results in a pause being heard in the regular pattern of the heart beat.

Contractility is the ability of the cardiac muscle cells to respond to a stimulus by shortening their fibres. To produce an efficient pumping action, the cardiac muscle fibres need to contract simultaneously. The force generated from this contraction is dependent on oxygen levels and an optimum balance of electrolytes, particularly calcium ions. Other factors affecting the contractile nature of cardiac cells include the effects of heart disease and medications (Dienhart et al 1984, p 16; Hanisch 1993, p 15).

THE HEART'S CONDUCTION SYSTEM

The normal conduction system of the heart follows an orderly pattern as seen in Figure 1.5. It comprises the SA node which is located in the right atrium close to the entry of the superior vena cava. This specialised bundle of cells, called *pacemaker cells*, is able to initiate impulses spontaneously at the rate of 60–100 bpm. The impulse is transmitted to the surrounding atrial muscles by another specialised group of cells known as myocardial working cells. There is some thought (though controversial) that the impulse leaves the SA node and is transmitted via three internodal pathways across the right atrium. These are the anterior, the middle (Wenckebach's bundle) and the posterior (Thorel's pathway) internodal tracts. An interatrial tract, called Bachman's bundle, branches off from the anterior nodal tract to the left atrium. The three internodal tracts converge at the AV node. It is not so much this node which is responsible for the transmission of electrical

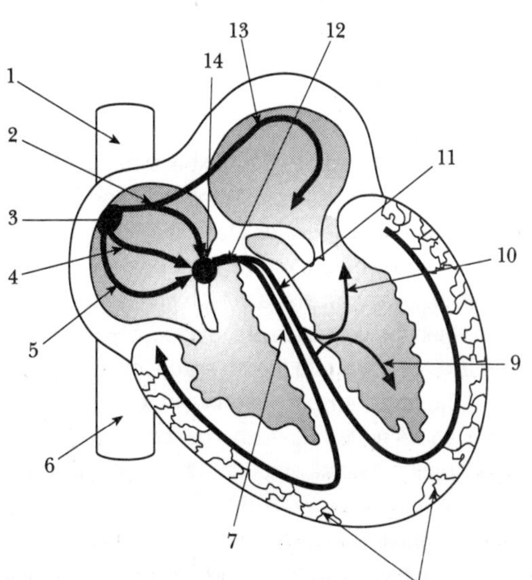

1 Superior vena cava
2 Anterior internodal tract
3 Sinoatrial (SA) node
4 Middle internodal tract (Wenckebach's bundle)
5 Posterior internodal tract (Thorel's pathway)
6 Inferior vena cava
7 Right bundle branch
8 Purkinje fibres
9 Anterior descending fascicle
10 Posterior descending fascicle
11 Left bundle branch
12 Bundle of His
13 Bachman's bundle (interatrial tract)
14 Atrioventricular (AV) node

FIGURE 1.5 *The heart's conduction system*

impulses, but rather the tissue surrounding the AV node — the junctional area, hence the term junctional arrythmias (see Chapter 4).

Like the SA node, pacemaker cells are present in the junctional area and, if the SA node should fail to emit an impulse, these specialised cells can take over the role as pacemaker by initiating an impulse at a rate of 40–60 bpm. The impulse is usually delayed at the AV node for about 0.07–0.10 seconds to allow for atrial contraction to occur. Though the right atrium depolarises before the left atrium, atrial depolarisation as a whole should take less than 0.11 seconds. The impulse then passes from the AV node to the bundle of His and then into the right and left bundle branches which arise from the muscular portion of the interventricular septum. The right bundle branch is located at the right side of the septum and merges with the Purkinje fibres. The left bundle branch divides into two sub-branches or fascicles: (i) the anterior descending fascicle extends to the anterior section down the left side of the interventricular septum; and (ii) the posterior descending fascicle travels to the posterior section of the left ventricle before terminating in the Purkinje fibres (Underhill et al 1989, p 10). The impulse is then transmitted through the Purkinje cells which, like other specialised cells, are located on the main conduction pathway. The Purkinje cells are capable of emitting an impulse at the rate of 20–40 bpm if the SA node or the AV node fail to emit an impulse in the required time frame. Depolarisation occurs in both ventricles simultaneously, commencing at the apex of the heart and moving upwards to the base of the heart. Repolarisation of the ventricles commences in the opposite direction, that is, from the base of the heart and moving downwards to the apex of the heart.

CARDIAC HAEMODYNAMICS

THE CARDIAC CYCLE

The period from the beginning of one heart beat to the next is termed the *cardiac cycle.* It consists of a period of relaxation (diastole) when the heart fills with blood, followed by a period of contraction (systole) when blood is ejected from the ventricles. The pressure gradients enable blood to flow from one chamber to another. In physics, we learn that fluid flows from areas of high pressure to areas of lower pressure. During diastole when the ventricles are relaxed, the AV valves open and blood returning from the veins flows into the atria and into the ventricles. Towards the end of diastole, the atrial muscle contracts in response to an electrical stimulus discharged from the SA node. During this period of contraction, the pressure rises within the atria, forcing a small amount of blood into the ventricles — an extra 15–25% of the total volume (Guyton 1991, pp 101–2). The ventricles then respond to this same electrical stimulus by contracting. During this phase, the pressure within the ventricle rises, forcing the AV valves to close and prevents blood flowing back into the atria. The ventricular pressure continues to rise and when the pressure exceeds the pressure in the aorta and the pulmonary artery (at this point left ventricular pressure is approximately 80 mmHg and later in this phase it reaches a maximum pressure of 120 mmHg) the aortic and pulmonary valves open and the blood is ejected into the pulmonary artery and the aorta. Initially, the blood flow is rapid. According to Underhill et al (1989, p 58) 'up to two-thirds of the stroke volume is ejected in this 0.09 second period from the left ventricle'.

As the pressure equalises between the ventricles and their corresponding artery, the blood flow slows from the ventricle. With the onset of diastole, the ventricles relax once more, the pressure within the chambers decreases and the semilunar valves snap shut to prevent blood flowing back from the aorta and the pulmonary artery. As ventricular pressure continues to fall below that of the now rising atrial pressure, the AV valves open and the ventricles begin to fill, repeating the process.

Cardiac output is the amount of blood pumped into the aorta by the left ventricle each minute. Normal cardiac output is approximately 5 L/min, but this varies with the metabolic demands of the body, the individual's age and body size. According to Guyton (1991, p 221) cardiac output is 'frequently stated in terms of the cardiac index, that is, the cardiac output per square metre of body surface area'.

Cardiac output is controlled not so much by the heart, but by the amount of venous blood returning to the heart. Under the Frank-Starling law, if an increased quantity of blood flows into the heart, the walls of the heart's chambers stretch to accommodate this volume. As a result of this stretching, the cardiac muscle contracts with an increased force, emptying the chamber just as efficiently and in the same manner as it would with normal volumes of blood present. Therefore, any extra blood coming into the chamber is not held back and with the help of an increased heart rate is pumped out. The rise in heart rate is due to the effects of two phenomena. Firstly, as the right atrium is stretched, so is the sinus node. As a result its rhythm alters, increasing the heart rate by as much as 15%. Secondly, a nervous reflex, called the Bainbridge reflex, is activated when the increased volume of blood causes the right atrial walls to stretch. An impulse is then transmitted to the brain to increase the heart rate which returns the message to the heart via the sympathetic nervous system (Guyton 1991, pp 221–2).

Cardiac output is measured by the following equation:

cardiac output (CO) = stroke volume (SV) x heart rate (HR).

Stroke volume is the amount of blood ejected during ventricular contraction with each beat of the heart. In adults this is approximately 70 mL/beat. To be more specific, it is the difference in the amount of blood remaining in the ventricle at the end of diastole and the residual volume of blood remaining at the end of systole. *Heart rate, preload, afterload, compliance* and *contraction* all influence the stroke volume.

Heart rate refers to the number of times ventricles contract within one minute. The normal resting heart rate is 60–100 bpm.

Preload refers to the degree of stretch of myocardial fibres immediately prior to contraction. It is the volume contained inside the ventricle which influences the degree of stretch. The ability of myocardial fibres to stretch was first described by Frank Starling (Frank-Starling law). His description points out that muscle fibres can only stretch to a predetermined length. If they are stretched beyond that point then they cannot work as effectively, which decreases stroke volume and cardiac output. Myocardial fibres can be likened to an elastic band which, if stretched beyond its maximum elasticity, results in permanent distortion, rendering it incapable to perform its original task. Once the heart muscles have been over stretched from conditions such as volume overload secondary to valvular incompetence, or extensive muscle damage from a myocardial infarction, the heart will not be able to pump effectively.

Afterload refers to the amount of resistance with which the ventricles have to work against to effectively eject blood into the pulmonary or systemic circulation. Conditions such as increased peripheral vascular resistance and pulmonary oedema will increase afterload.

Compliance describes the extent to which the ventricle is capable of distending. To be more specific, compliance is a reflection of the amount of pressure within the ventricle immediately prior to systole. Compliance is also known as the left ventricular end-diastolic pressure. This pressure is the result of blood draining into the chamber from the left atrium during diastole. The compliance of the ventricle can alter as a consequence of longstanding heart disease or damage to the muscle, as in the case of myocardial infarctions which cause the ventricle's compliance to decrease.

REFERENCES

Dienhart, C, Egoville, B, Honser, D, McCauley, K, Marker, C & Strong, A 1984, 'Understanding Fundamental Facts' in *Cardiovascular Disorders*, Nurses Clinical Library, Springhouse Corporation, Philadelphia

Gilchrist, B, Robertson, C, Webb, C & Wright, S 1992, *The Textbook of Adult Nursing*, adapted from Brunner, L & Suddarth, J (eds), *Lippincott Textbook of Medical and Surgical Nursing*, 6th edn, J B Lippincott Company, Philadelphia

Guyton, A 1991, *Textbook of Medical Physiology*, 8th edn, W B Saunders Company, Philadelphia

Hanisch, P 1993, 'Cardiac Anatomy and Physiology', in *Advanced Skills. Deciphering Difficult ECGs*, Springhouse Corporation, Philadelphia

Holloway, N 1993, *Nursing the Critically Ill Adult*, 4th edn, Addison-Wesley Publishing Co Inc, Redding

Ignatavicius, D & Bayne, M J 1991, *Medical–Surgical Nursing. A Nursing Process Approach*, W B Saunders Company, Philadelphia

Luckman, J & Sorenson, K 1987, *Medical and Surgical Nursing. A Psychophysiologic Approach*, W B Saunders Company, Philadelphia

Oh, T E 1990, *Intensive Care Manual,* 3rd edn, Butterworths, Sydney

Smeltzer, S & Bare, B 1992, *Brunner and Suddarth's Textbook of Medical Surgical Nursing*, 7th edn, J B Lippincott Company, Philadelphia

Underhill, S, Woods, S, Froelicher, E and Halpenny, C 1989, *Cardiac Nursing*, 2nd edn, J B Lippincott Company, Philadelphia

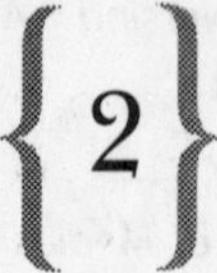

ELECTROCARDIOGRAPHY

OBJECTIVES

After working through this chapter you should be able to:

- define electrocardiography
- describe and discuss the principles of electrocardiography
- identify the deflections, segments and intervals of a normal ECG complex
- relate the ECG complex to the events of the cardiac cycle
- recognise normal sinus rhythm
- describe the steps involved to interpret cardiac rhythms

KEY WORDS

bipolar lead
ECG complex
electrical axis
electrocardiogram
electrocardiography
heart rate
isoelectric line
J point
P wave
PR interval
precordial lead
QRS complex
QT interval
rhythm
ST segment
T wave
unipolar lead
wave deflection

ELECTROCARDIOGRAPHY

Electrocardiography is the means by which the electrical potential generated by cardiac cells during a cardiac cycle can be graphically recorded using an electrocardiograph (ECG) machine. As a wave of electrical energy travels along the heart's conduction system, electrodes placed on specific sites of the patient's skin sense the electrical activity and transmit the details to the recording equipment. Inside the ECG machine a device called a galvanometer interprets the current of electricity and amplifies the current. With the assistance of a hot stylus or an ink pen (depending on the make and the model of the ECG machine), the ECG machine records the electrical activity as a series of upward and downward deflections onto moving graph paper. This printed record is called an *electrocardiogram* or *ECG* (Dubin 1989; Meltzer, Pinneo & Kitchell 1983).

'ECG' is often used to describe the special graph paper used to record the electrocardiogram, the recording machines, the actual procedure, the printed record from a full 12 lead and the printed record from a single monitoring lead.

A number of procedures are used to record the heart's electrical pattern. Some of these are:

1 12 lead electrocardiography
2 continuous cardiac monitoring
3 ambulatory monitoring (using a Holter monitor)
4 exercise electrocardiography (stress testing)
5 telemetry monitoring
6 electrophysiological studies (EPS).

With the exception of 12 lead electrocardiography, the above procedures will be discussed in more detail in Chapter 3.

ELECTROCARDIOGRAPH PAPER

The ECG is recorded on special graph paper which contains ruled lines which are 1 mm apart on the horizontal and the vertical axes. The graph paper moves from the ECG machine normally at the rate of 25 mm/sec, however there are times during the recording of a single lead when the operator may decide to change the paper rate to 50 mm/sec to allow for better visualisation of individual waves.

Before any recording takes place, it is important to standardise the ECG. This is achieved by pressing the '1 mV' button on the ECG machine.

The height of the ensuing 1 mV trace on the graph paper is 10 mm which is equal to two large squares (see Figure 2.1). This standardisation or calibration mark assists in accurately interpretating the ECG. In the presence of some cardiac conditions, for example left ventricular hypertrophy (enlargement of the left ventricle), the standardisation factor may have to be reduced to 0.5 so the wave amplitude of the QRS complex remains on the graph paper. At this factor the 1 mV trace is only 5 mm high.

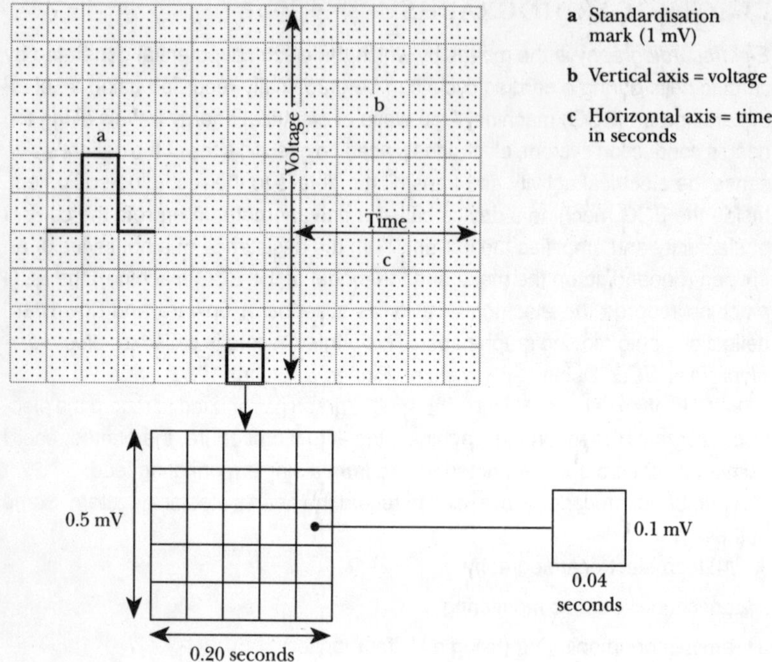

FIGURE 2.1 *ECG paper*

If the wave amplitude is very small the standardisation factor may have to be increased to 2 to enhance its visibility. At this factor the 1 mV trace is 20 mm high.

It is important to ensure that the standardisation factor is marked on the graph paper to assist the practitioner in reaching the correct interpretation.

When recording the ECG it is important that the ECG wave forms are produced with a standardisation factor that maximises the wave amplitude while keeping all the waves on the graph paper. Failure to do this may result in inaccurate or incomplete interpretations and may result in repeating the procedure.

The **vertical axis** on the graph paper measures **voltage**. For example, when standardising the ECG at 1 mV for a 10 mm high trace, each millimetre space represents 0.1 mV. Therefore, each 5 mm space between heavy lines represents 0.5 mV (see Figure 2.1).

The **horizontal axis** measures **time** in seconds. Each millimetre space represents 0.04 seconds, therefore the distance between two heavy dark lines or 5 mm is equivalent to 0.20 seconds (see Figure 2.1).

These basic measurements of time and voltage are important to understand and remember as they are used in cardiac rhythm interpretation. Time measurement is used to indicate alterations in conduction times of the wave forms representing depolarisation and repolarisation. Voltage measurement results in changes in strength and direction of the wave forms.

THE ELECTROCARDIOGRAM

To obtain a recording of the heart's electrical activity on ECG paper, electrodes — suction cups, small metal plates or the disposable paper variety — need to be placed in specific anatomical positions on the patient's body (see Figure 2.2).

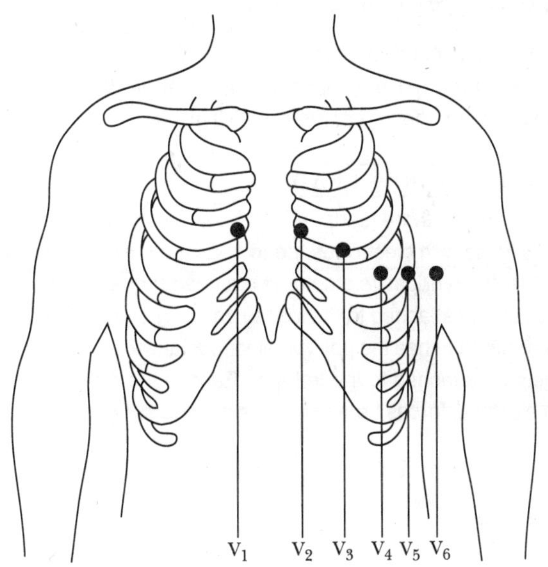

FIGURE 2.2 *Position of electrodes for a 12 lead ECG*

Since the heart's electrical activity travels in many directions, using 12 leads (and sometimes more) enables this pattern to be viewed from a variety of angles. Together with the patient's clinical history and specific blood tests, the ECG detects and interprets any injury, disease or infection to the cardiac tissue. This information is used to determine how the patient will be managed. The data supplied by an electrocardiogram includes:

- disorders of the heart beat (rate and rhythm)
- conduction defects (time delays between the SA node and the AV node, for example, first degree AV block)
- damage to the myocardium, for example, ischaemia, infarction, infection
- atrial and ventricular hypertrophy

- electrolyte imbalances, for example, hyperkalaemia, hypokalaemia
- effects of drug intoxication, for example, digoxin, quinidine.

Like other assessment tools, ECGs have their limitations. For example, they cannot determine when a myocardial infarction will actually occur and, even though ischaemic heart disease may be present in certain individuals, a resting ECG may not indicate that there is, in fact, an abnormality present. In addition, an ECG cannot provide information pertaining to cardiac output.

LEADS AND THEIR POSITIONS

The term *lead* refers to the difference in electrical potential between a pair of electrodes. There are three types of leads: *bipolar (standard) leads*, *unipolar (augmented) leads* and the *chest (precordial* or *'V') leads*.

BIPOLAR (STANDARD) LEADS

In this arrangement the three leads — lead I, lead II and lead III — are attached to the patient's limbs with electrodes. **Lead I** has the positive electrode attached to the left arm and the negative electrode attached to the right arm. **Lead II** has the positive electrode attached to the left leg and the negative electrode attached to the right arm. **Lead III** has the positive electrode attached to the left leg and the negative electrode attached to the left arm. Each of the three leads records the difference in electrical forces between two electrode sites.

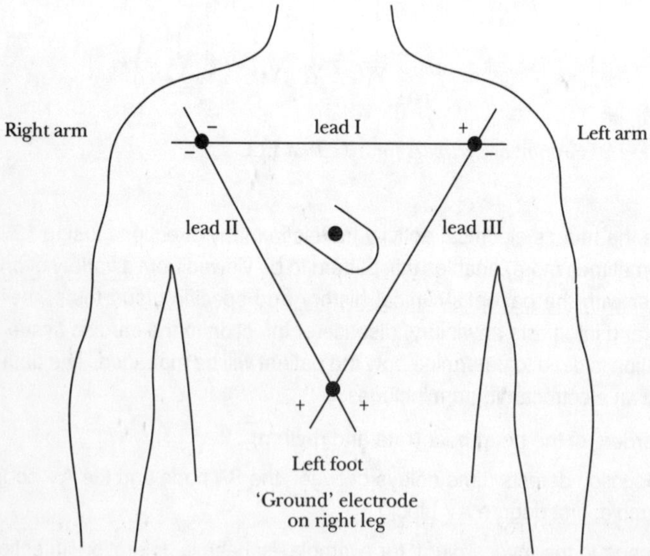

FIGURE 2.3 *Bipolar leads*

By drawing lines to connect each of the electrodes, an equilateral triangle is formed around the heart and is referred to as *Einthoven's triangle* (see Figure 2.4).

Einthoven's principle states that if the electrical potentials of any two bipolar electrodes are known at any given instant, the third electrical potential can be calculated as the sum of the first two.

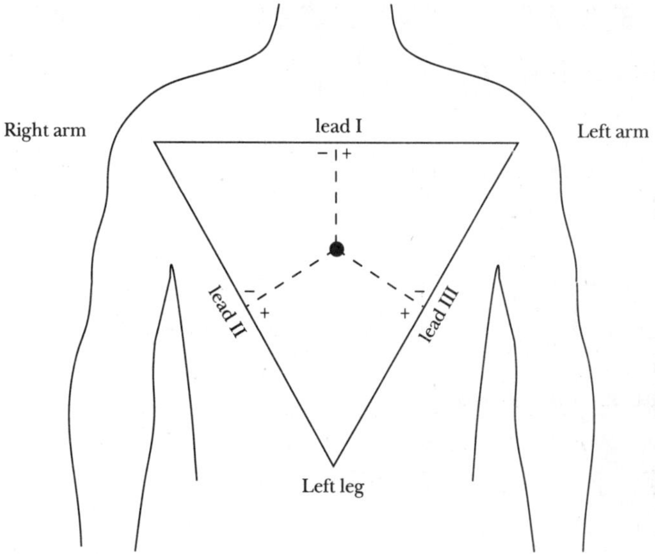

FIGURE 2.4 *Einthoven's triangle*

Source Adapted from Underhill et al 1989, p 310

UNIPOLAR (AUGMENTED) LEADS

In this arrangement one positive electrode is placed on each of the following limbs: right arm, left arm and left foot. These leads measure the electrical potential between the centre of the heart and each limb (see Figure 2.5).

aV_R = the positive electrode on the right arm. **aV_L** = the positive electrode on the left arm. **aV_F** = the positive electrode on the left foot.

An electrode placed on the right leg completes the circuit and acts as the 'ground' electrode. Together, the bipolar and the unipolar leads view the heart using the vertical axis.

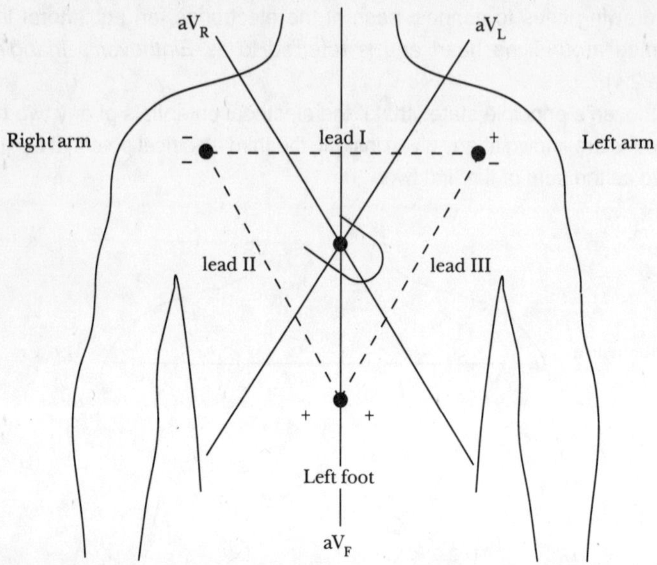

FIGURE 2.5 *Unipolar leads*

CHEST (PRECORDIAL) LEADS

Unipolar leads have six positive electrodes which view the left ventricle using the horizontal axis (see Figure 2.6). However, if more information is required about the right ventricle, electrodes can be placed in the identical positions on the right side of the chest. Placement of the electrodes is as follows.

V_1 — on the right side of the sternum at the fourth intercostal space
V_2 — on the left side of the sternum at the fourth intercostal space
V_3 — midway between **V_2** and **V_4**
V_4 — on the mid-clavicular line at the fifth intercostal space
V_5 — on the anterior axillary line, horizontal to **V_4**
V_6 — on the mid-axillary line, horizontal to **V_4** and **V_5**

Together, leads I, II, III, aV_R, aV_L, aV_F, V_1, V_2, V_3, V_4, V_5 and V_6 generate a 12 lead ECG which resembles that shown in Figure 2.7 on page 22.

WAVE DEFLECTIONS

When viewing a 12 lead ECG, the P waves, QRS complex and the T wave are positive, that is, above the baseline or the isoelectric line (the straight line which forms the PR interval and the ST segment) in some leads, and negative, or below

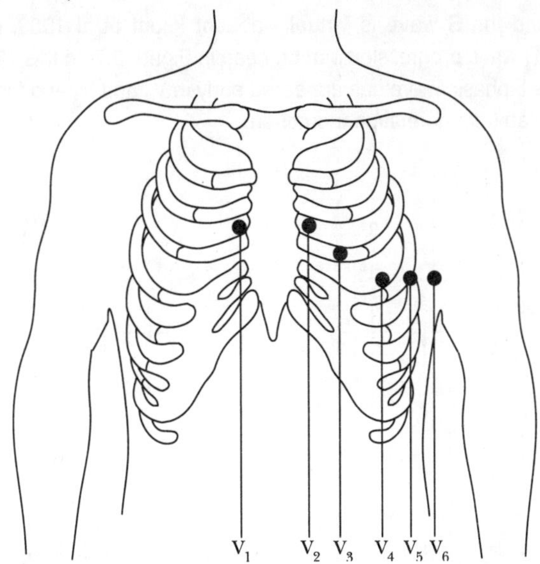

FIGURE 2.6 *Location of the chest leads*

the baseline, in other leads. You will notice, too, that the QRS complex in V_3 and V_4 is biphasic, that is, half the wave is above the baseline and the other half of the wave is below the baseline.

DIFFERENCES IN WAVE DEFLECTIONS

If a positive electrode is placed in the path of an oncoming wave of electrical activity, for example during depolarisation, the deflection (or direction) of the P wave, QRS complex and T wave will be positive (or pointing upwards from the isoelectric line). The chest leads — V_5 and V_6 — are examples of this deflection (see Figure 2.8). However, if the electrode is not facing the wave of electrical activity, as with aV_R, V_1 and V_2, the P wave, the QRS complex and the T wave will have mostly negative deflections (or point downwards from the isoelectric line).

The biphasic wave pattern observed in V_3 and V_4 is due to the fact that these leads are placed over the septum and the wave of electrical activity is at right angles to the leads.

The relationship between the direction of the heart's electrical activity and the position of a positive electrode is demonstrated clearly in the chest (V) leads. Normally, in V_1 the QRS complex is negative, but sometimes there can be a small R wave present. In V_2 the R wave becomes slightly more positive; in V_3 and V_4 the proportion of R wave to S wave is about equal; and in V_5 and V_6 the R wave is upright and the S wave is virtually absent (Hunt et al 1983, p 100). An example of R wave progression can be seen in Figure 2.7. In this 12 lead ECG note that the biphasic wave has appeared early in V_2 and V_3 and for some individuals this can be a normal phenomenon.

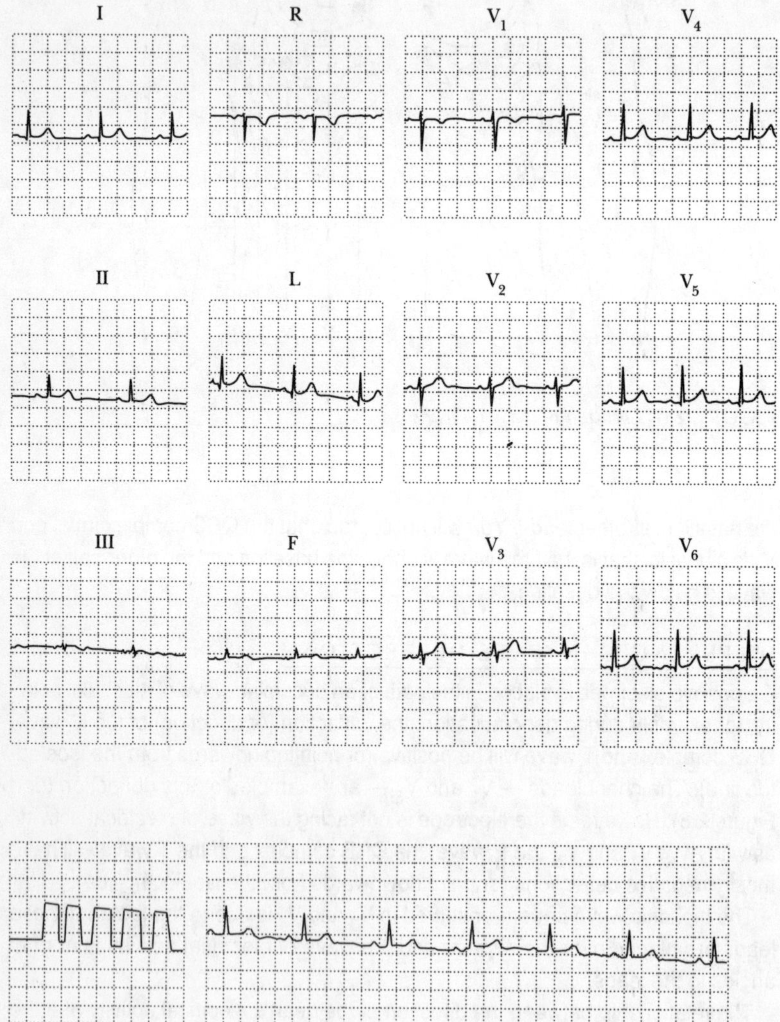

FIGURE 2.7 *Normal 12 lead ECG*

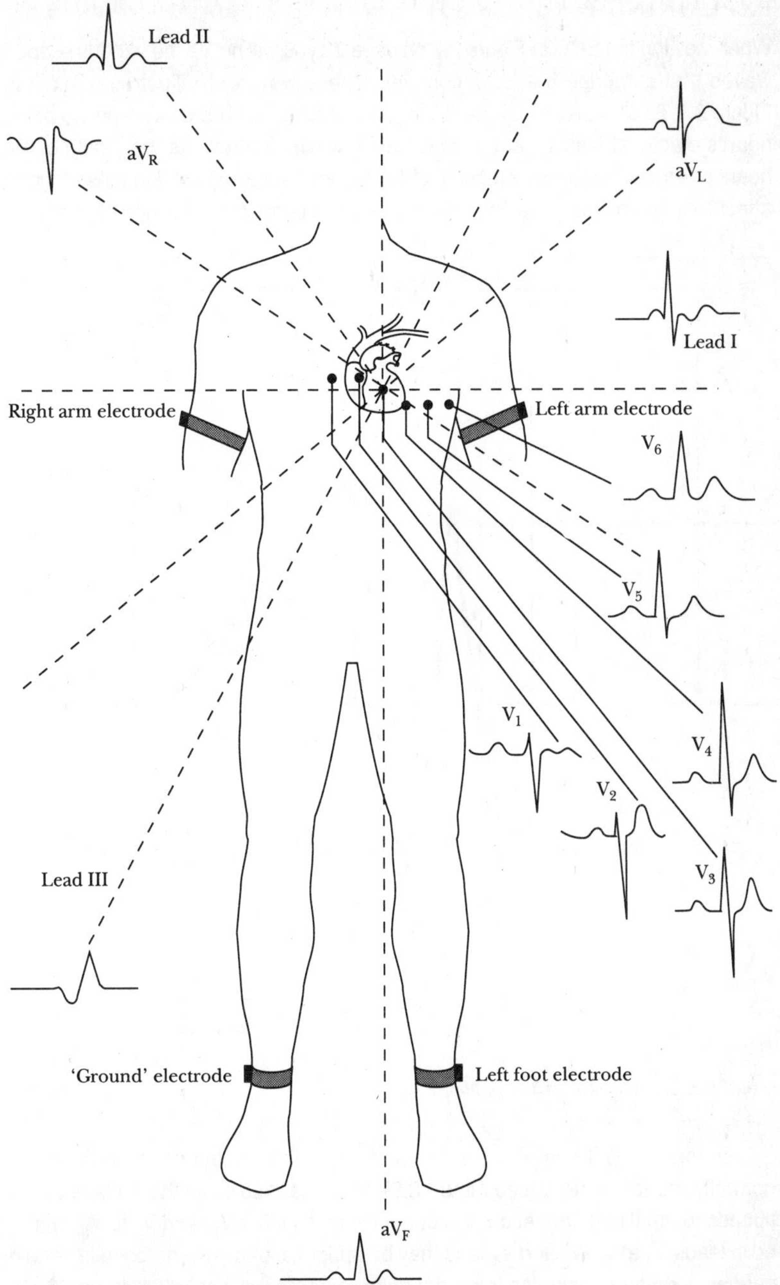

FIGURE 2.8 *Normal wave deflections*

EXPLAINING P, Q, R, S & T

When viewing the ECG in Figure 2.7 on page 22 you will notice the various shaped waves that comprise the ECG complex. These waves are illustrated again in Figure 2.8. Each wave is important, not just because they represent a phase of the heart's electrical activity, but because each wave also reflects the health of the heart in terms of disease, infection and injury and the way in which these factors affect initiation of impulses and their subsequent conduction through the heart.

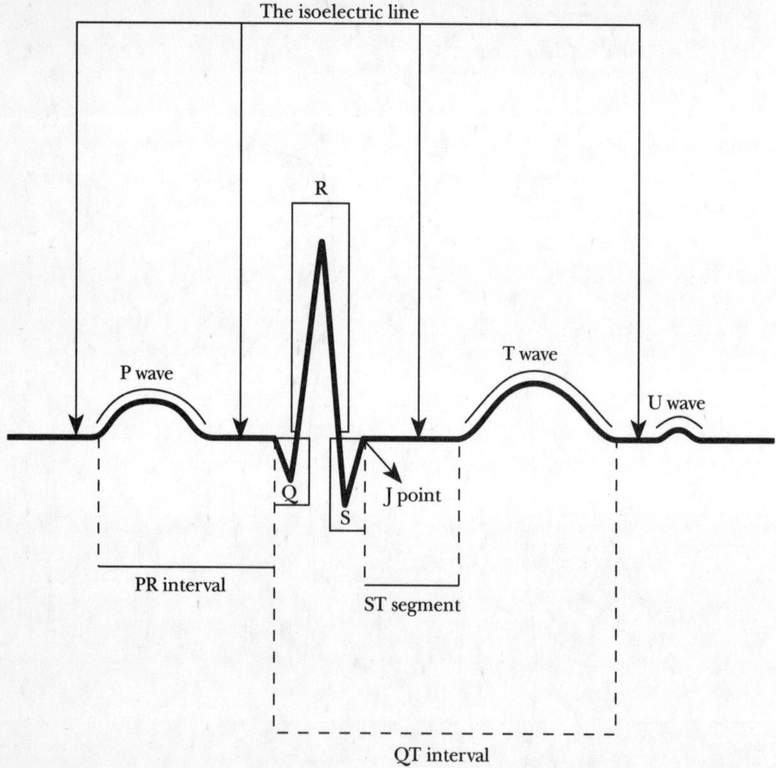

FIGURE 2.9 *Normal ECG complex*

In a normal ECG complex the first upright wave is called the *P wave* and is normally round in shape (see Figure 2.9). In the cardiac cycle the P wave corresponds to atrial depolarisation. It is upright in leads I, II, aV_F, and V_2 to V_6; inverted in leads III, aV_R aV_L and V_1; and may be upright, biphasic or notched in certain cardiac conditions, such as left atrial enlargement (see Table 2.1 on pp 26–7). The height of the P wave should not exceed 3 mm in the bipolar leads and

2.5 mm in the unipolar leads when the ECG has been standardised at 10 mm deflection for 1 mV.

The isoelectric line following the P wave forms part of the *PR interval* which is measured from the beginning of the P wave to the beginning of the QRS complex. If there is a Q wave present, the PR interval is measured up to the start of this wave. If there is no Q wave present, the PR interval is measured up to the start of the R wave. The PR interval represents the time between activation of the sinus node and the impulse spreading across the atria to the ventricular muscle. It is normally 0.10–0.20 seconds (2.5–5 mm) in length.

The *Q wave* is the first downward or negative deflection below the isoelectric line following the P wave and, as discussed earlier, may or may not be present. If present, its depth should not exceed 25% of the R wave.

The R wave follows the Q wave and is easily recognised as the first upward deflection after the P wave. The S wave is the next downward deflection. Together, these three waves form the *QRS complex* and represent ventricular depolarisation which normally measures 0.08–0.12 seconds (2–3 mm) in length. The bulk of the QRS complex has a positive deflection in leads I, II, aV_L, aV_F, V_5 and V_6. It is mostly negative in leads III, aV_R, V_1 and V_2 and may be biphasic in V_3 and V_4.

Like the P wave, the QRS complex has a variety of shapes which often result from disease, infection, trauma and the position of the heart within the chest cavity (see Table 2.1).

The *ST segment* is the isoelectric line between the end of the QRS complex and the beginning of the T wave and represents early ventricular repolarisation. The point where the S wave meets the ST segment is referred to as the *J point.*

Under certain cardiac conditions, the ST segment may be depressed (below the baseline), as in myocardial ischaemia, or elevated (above the baseline), as with pericarditis or a myocardial infarction (MI). For the elevation to be significant it must be at least 2 mm high. Normally, depression of the ST segment should not be greater than 0.5 mm. Variations in the shape of the ST segment are illustrated in Table 2.1.

The *T wave* is the rounded upright wave following the ST segment and represents repolarisation of the ventricles. In some of the leads of the 12 lead ECG, the appearance of the T wave may alter. For instance, it is always inverted in aV_R and may be inverted or upright in leads III, aV_L, aV_F, V_1 and V_2. In the limb leads the height of the T wave should not exceed 5 mm and in the precordial (chest) leads it should not be greater than 10 mm in height.

However, under certain conditions, such as in the presence of hyperkalaemia (elevated serum potassium), tall peaked T waves will be observed on the cardiac trace. Deep symmetrically inverted T waves may be seen in the presence of myocardial ischaemia or an evolving MI. Variations in the shape of the T wave are illustrated in Table 2.1.

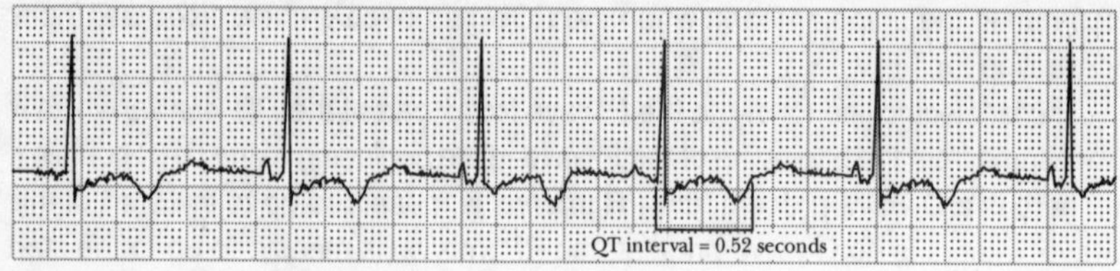

FIGURE 2.10 *Effects of amiodarone on the QT interval*

The *QT interval* represents electrical systole and is measured from the beginning of the Q wave (or the R wave if the Q wave is absent) to the end of the T wave. The QT interval varies in accordance with the patient's heart rate, their age and sex. Normally, the QT interval should be 0.32–0.40 seconds if the heart rate is 70 bpm. When the heart rate varies, the QT interval needs to be corrected using a nomogram (Underhill et al 1989, p 313).

Lengthening of the QT interval (greater than 0.42 seconds) may be caused by conditions such as myocarditis, myocardial ischaemia or the effects of anti-arrhythmic agents, which include quinidine, procainamide and amiodarone (see Figure 2.10); psychotrophic medications, which include tricyclic antidepressants, and electrolyte disturbances (hypokalaemia, hypocalcaemia and hypomagnesium). Neurological trauma, such as a subarachnoid haemorrhage, may also extend the duration of the QT interval.

Normal wave shape	Alterations in shape	Possible implications
P wave	Inverted	Normally this shape appears in some of the chest and limb leads
	Notched	Quinidine toxicity
	Diphasic	Atrial enlargement
	Flattened	Hyperkalaemia
	Diphasic	Right atrial enlargement
	Diphasic	Left atrial enlargement
QRS complex	Rabbit's ear pattern	Right bundle branch block, visualised in lead V_1
	Broad and notched	Left bundle branch block, visualised in lead V_6
	Pathological Q wave	Q wave, one third of the height of R wave and 0.04 seconds in width. Associated with MI

Cont next page

Normal wave shape	Alterations in shape	Possible implications
QRS complex 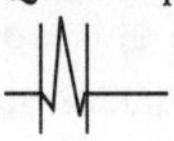	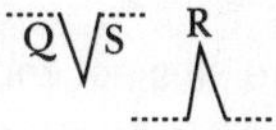 Q S R	Lead positioning in some limb or chest leads
ST segment 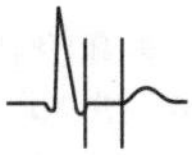	(i) 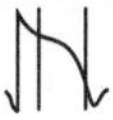	ST segment elevation associated with injury to myocardium
	(ii) 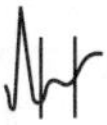	Non-Q wave infarction Exercise induced ischaemia
	(iii) 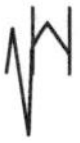 or 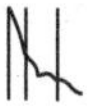	Flat or concave elevated ST segment in pericarditis
		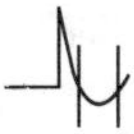 Effects of digoxin therapy
T wave 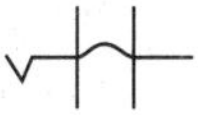	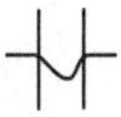 Assymetrically inverted	Left ventricular hypertrophy
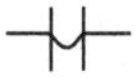	Inverted	Myocardial ischaemia
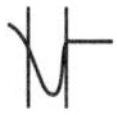	Deep symmetrical T wave.	Evolving MI
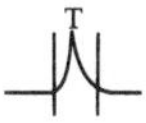	T Peaked T wave	Hyperkalaemia
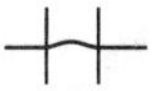	Flat T wave	Hypokalaemia
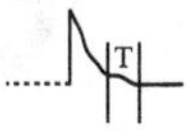	T Elevated T wave	Associated with pericarditis

TABLE 2.1 *Variations in the shape of the waves and segments of the ECG complex*

Excessively prolonged QT intervals are associated with a life-threatening form of ventricular tachycardia (see Chapter 4 for further discussion) called *Torsades de Pointes* translated as dancing on the points, that is, the heart's electrical axis continually alters.

The *U wave* sometimes follows the T wave. It is not known whether it represents the end of ventricular repolarisation, but it is prominent in conditions such as hypokalaemia.

THE HEART'S ELECTRICAL AXIS

Dubin (1978, p 150) describes the heart's electrical axis as the direction (represented by a vector) in which the wave of depolarisation moves throughout the heart. When the electrical impulse is initiated from the SA node, hundreds of vectors are formed. The vectors travel in different directions and many tend to cancel out one another, forming a mean QRS vector. The mean QRS vector normally points down from the AV node and to the left side of the patient's chest because that is where the bulk of ventricular tissue lies.

To locate the exact position of the mean QRS vector a circle, divided into four quadrants, is drawn over the patient's chest (see Figure 2.11). The lower half of

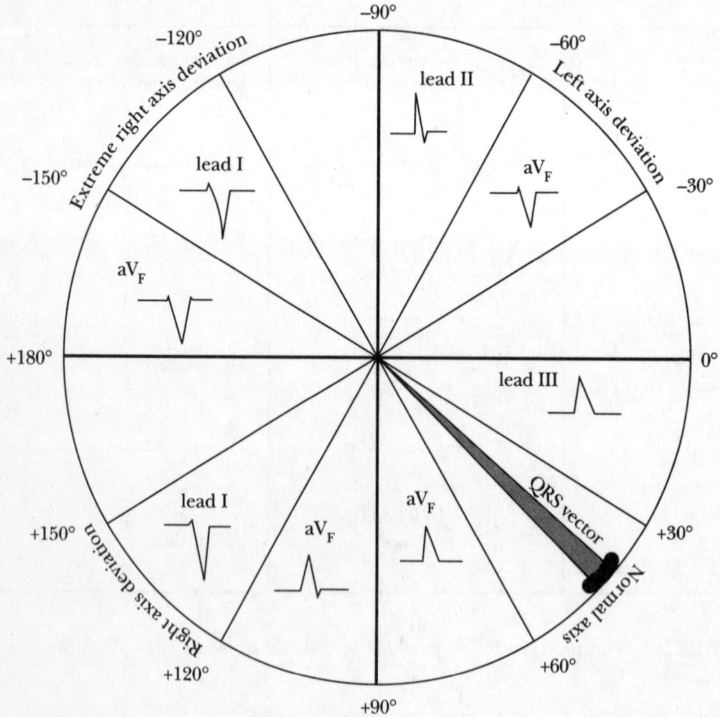

FIGURE 2.11 *The heart's electrical axis*

Source Adapted from Dubin 1978, p 156

the circle in Figure 2.11 is divided into degrees ranging from 0 to +180° and the upper half of the circle ranges from –180 to 0°.

As the normal axis points downward and to the left, the mean QRS vector should be located within the 0 to +90° range.

However, opinions differ as to what constitutes the range for normal axis deviation. Authors such as Holloway (1993, p 303) and Julian (1984, p 47) use the range –30 to +110° for the heart's normal electrical axis. Sheidt (1986, p 3) suggests that the normal axis may fall in the range of +90 to +105° and –15 to –30°.

Chronic cardiac disease, for example, left ventricular hypertrophy, or the lie of the heart in the patient's chest cause the axis to deviate to the left or to the right. In left axis deviation, the mean QRS vector points into the upper right quadrant (–90 to 0°) and in right axis deviation, the resultant QRS vector is located in the range +90 to +150° (see Figure 2.11).

To calculate whether there is left or right axis deviation, only the limb leads — leads I and aV_F — are selected from the 12 lead ECG.

Left axis deviation — the QRS complex is positive (points upwards from the isoelectric line) in lead I and is negative in aV_F.

Right axis deviation — the QRS complex is negative in lead I and positive in aV_F.

Extreme right axis deviation — (–180 to –90°) the QRS complex is negative in lead I and negative in aV_F.

INTERPRETING THE CARDIAC RHYTHM

The cardiac rhythm provides information about the condition of the conduction system in terms of the location of the initial impulse, whether it be in the SA node, the atrial walls, junctional area,or the ventricular pathways. The cardiac rhythm also provides information about the subsequent conduction route, the time it takes for the impulse to accomplish its journey and whether or not it is regular. In healthy adults, the normal cardiac rhythm is called *sinus rhythm* because the site of the initial impulse arises in the SA node. Each minute a regular impulse is emitted at the rate of 60–100 bpm when the person is resting. Naturally, this rate changes according to the metabolic demands of the body. For example, during exercise, the heart rate will exceed 100 bpm, but when the individual stops and rests, the heart rate will return to its normal range.

After the impulse leaves the SA node it travels through the normal conduction pathway without any delay. Therefore, sinus rhythm is characterised by the following features:

- regular rhythm
- a heart rate within the normal range of 60–100 bpm
- normal P waves which precede the QRS complex

- a PR interval which is in the normal range of 0.12–0.20 seconds in duration
- a QRS complex which measures from 0.06 to 0.12 seconds.

Examples of normal sinus rhythm are illustrated in Figure 2.12.

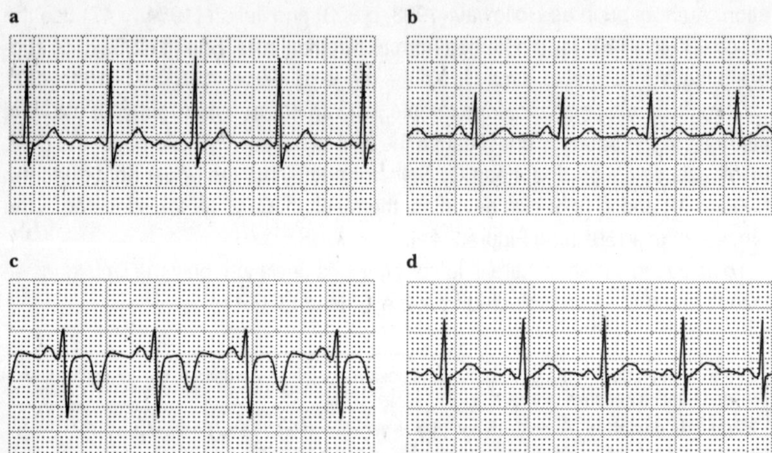

FIGURE 2.12 *Examples of normal sinus rhythm*

When the rate, rhythm or conduction pattern of a cardiac rhythm fails to meet the normal criteria, the resulting disorder is termed an *arrhythmia*.

According to their disorder arrhythmias are classified into two main groups. The first group of arrhythmias is due to **disorders in impulse formation**. The SA node is the heart's pacemaker which discharges a regular impulse at the rate of 60–100 bpm. However, under certain conditions the SA node may fail to emit an impulse, or the impulse may arise from outside the SA node, for example, in the atrial walls, in the tissue surrounding the AV node (junctional area), or from within the ventricle. Depending on where the site of impulse formation arises, and whether there is any underlying pathology present, this will determine the rate and pattern of subsequent impulses discharged, for example atrial fibrillation. This arrhythmia can arise as a result of atrial enlargement. In this condition, the muscle walls become irritated from being overstretched and discharge impulses from multiple sites at a rate in excess of 350 bpm, overriding the SA node. The pattern displayed on the cardiac monitor shows an irregular rhythm characterised by a wavy baseline with no discernible P waves.

There are four main types of rhythm:

1 **Bradycardia** In this regular rhythm the ventricular heart rate is between 40 and 60 bpm (eg sinus bradycardia).

2 **Tachycardia** This is a regular rhythm exceeding 100 bpm. An exception to this is sinus tachycardia which has an upper rate limit of 150 bpm. However, under certain conditions (eg an athlete participating in strenuous physical activity), this upper limit may be exceeded, but it should not be greater than 200 bpm. Ventricular tachycardia may often exceed 200 bpm.

3 **Flutter** This is a regular rhythm with a saw tooth appearance (eg atrial flutter). For more information on flutter rhythm, refer to Chapter 4.

4 **Fibrillation** This is characterised by an irregular, chaotic and wavy baseline in which some or most of the complexes comprising the ECG complex cannot be clearly visualised (eg ventricular fibrillation; Holloway 1993, p 308). Refer to Chapter 4 for greater detail of ventricular fibrillation.

The second classification system for arrhythmia identification relates to those patterns where there is a **delay or a block in the conduction of the impulses**. Delays occur in the SA node. Examples of this include sinoatrial block; between the atria and the ventricles — first degree AV block; and within the ventricles — left bundle branch block.

In order to obtain a clear picture of the patient's cardiac rhythm, most health care facilities use lead II as the preferred monitoring lead because the QRS complex can be seen more clearly and the P wave is upright. Samples of the patient's cardiac rhythm can be obtained from the strip recorder on the cardiac monitor or during the recording of a 12 lead ECG. If the sample is collected from the cardiac monitor, it should measure at least 150–200 mm in length. (See Chapter 3 for further discussion on monitoring leads and the cardiac monitor.)

To master the art of cardiac rhythm interpretation it is important to use a systematic method and to practise the skill as much as possible. At times, some of the rhythms can be difficult to interpret and it will be necessary to seek further assistance from an individual who is skilled in cardiac rhythm interpretation.

The method introduced here for interpreting the cardiac rhythm involves eight steps discussed below.

IS THE CARDIAC RHYTHM REGULAR?

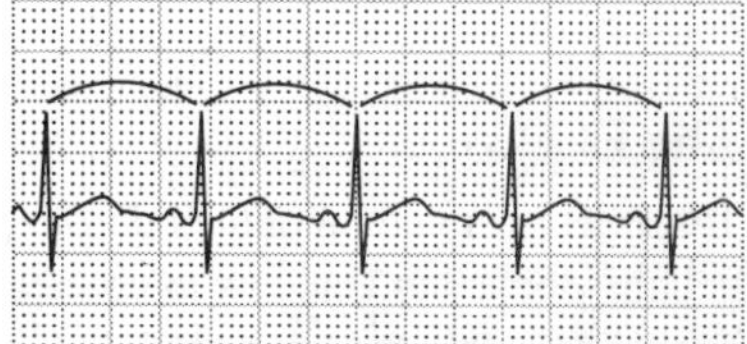

FIGURE 2.13a (left) *Irregular cardiac rhythm*
FIGURE 2.13b (right) *Regular cardiac rhythm*

To determine the regularity of the cardiac rhythm the easiest method is to look at the rhythm and see if it appears regular. Figure 2.13 on page 31 shows examples of an irregular and a regular cardiac rhythm. In some cardiac rhythm traces (like the examples shown), it is obvious whether or not the rhythm is regular. However, in others it is not clear and for this reason this method can have its limitations.

If you are unsure of the regularity of the cardiac rhythm, take a blank piece of paper and place the uppermost edge near the top of the R waves. Using a pencil, mark on the paper two R waves. Then move the paper along to the next two R waves and see if the previous two marks on the paper coincide with these waves. Continue to do this until you reach the end of the trace. This method of determining the regularity of a cardiac rhythm is demonstrated in Figure 2.14.

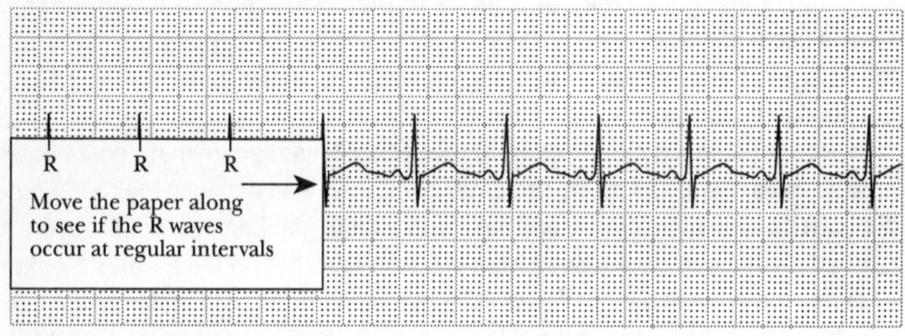

FIGURE 2.14 *Determining the regularity of a cardiac rhythm*

WHAT IS THE HEART RATE?

To calculate the heart rate, a number of approaches can be used. Today, cardiac monitors and ECG machines automatically record the heart rate at the top of the cardiac rhythm strip. However, this function may not always be available and sometimes when the wave amplitude is small or there is extraneous interference, for example when a patient is cleaning their teeth, the rate documented can be grossly inaccurate.

The ECG ruler

The ECG ruler can be obtained from pharmaceutical companies who distribute antiarrhythmic medications to hospital pharmacy departments. Using the ECG ruler to calculate the heart rate is a particularly useful method when the rhythm under examination is regular and the rate is less than 60 bpm. There are two sides to the ruler, each marked according to the paper speed being used (see Figure 2.15).

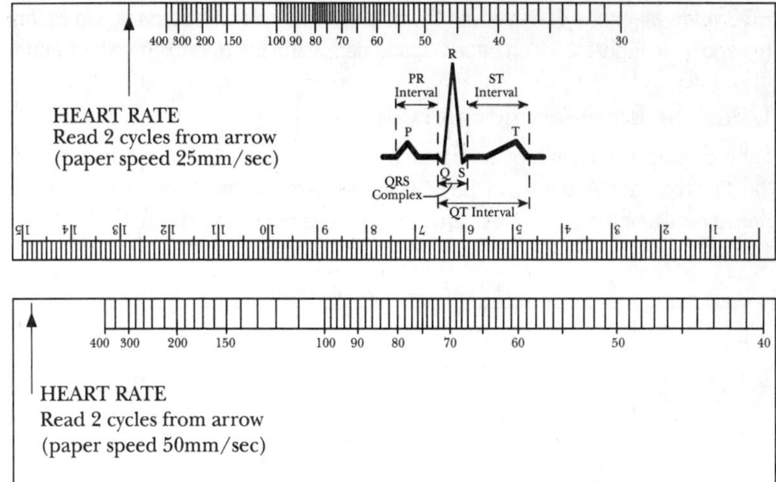

FIGURE 2.15 *ECG ruler*

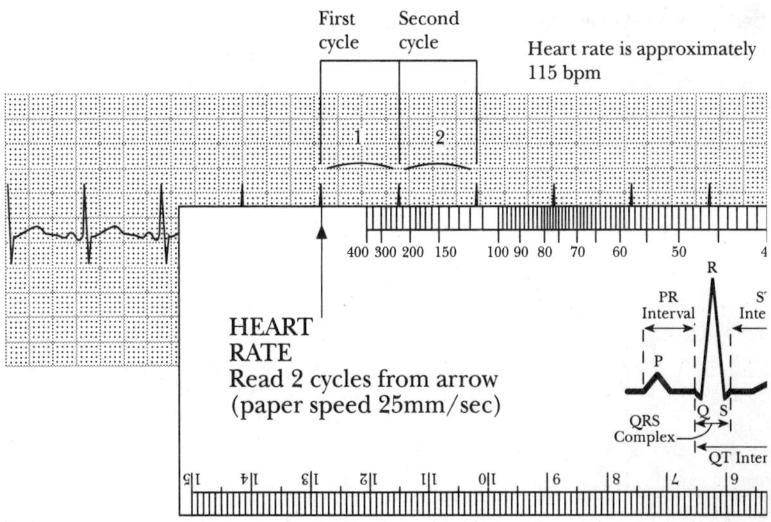

FIGURE 2.16 *Calculating the heart rate using the ECG ruler.*

To use the ruler, determine the paper speed which will be set on the cardiac monitor or the ECG machine (normally 25 mm/sec). Using the appropriate side of the

ECG ruler, align one R wave with the arrow on the ruler. Read back two cycles (as shown in Figure 2.16 on page 33) and determine the approximate heart rate.

Using the three-second intervals

If the cardiac rhythm is regular, obtain a sample trace of 200 mm in length from the strip recorder. At the top of the ECG paper there are small vertical lines occurring at regular intervals — these are the three-second intervals (see Figure 2.17).

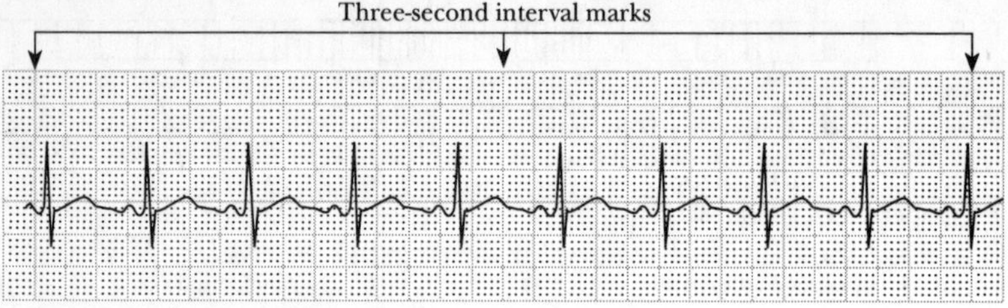

FIGURE 2.17 *Calculating the heart rate using the three-second intervals*

To calculate the heart rate, take two three-second intervals and count the number of R waves which fall in six seconds. (From the first three-second mark to the next equals three seconds and from the second three-second mark to the third equals three seconds — a total of six seconds.) Next, multiply the number of R waves by 10 and this will yield an approximate ventricular rate per minute. The same technique can be utilised for calculating the atrial rate (see Figure 2.18).

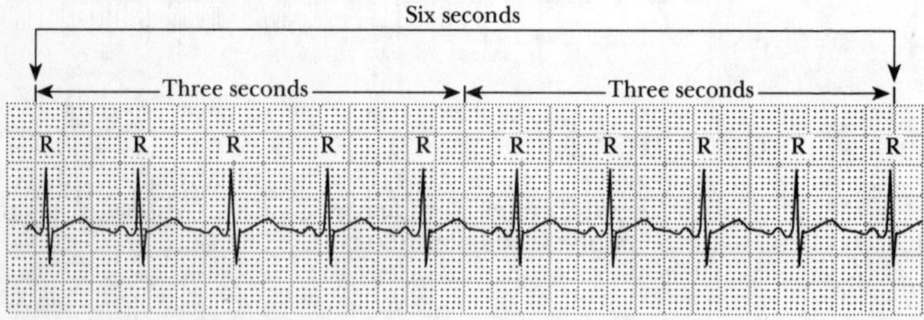

FIGURE 2.18 *Calculating the heart rate using the R waves. In the above example there are 10 R waves in the six-second strip. Therefore 10 × 10 = 100 and the ventricular heart rate is approximately 100 bpm.*

Alternatively, if the rhythm is irregular, some authors (Underhill et al 1989, p 314; Dubin 1978, pp 68–70) suggest that a more accurate method of estimating the heart rate can be made by counting the number of RR cycles in six seconds and multiplying this figure by 10 to yield an approximate heart rate per minute (see Figure 2.19).

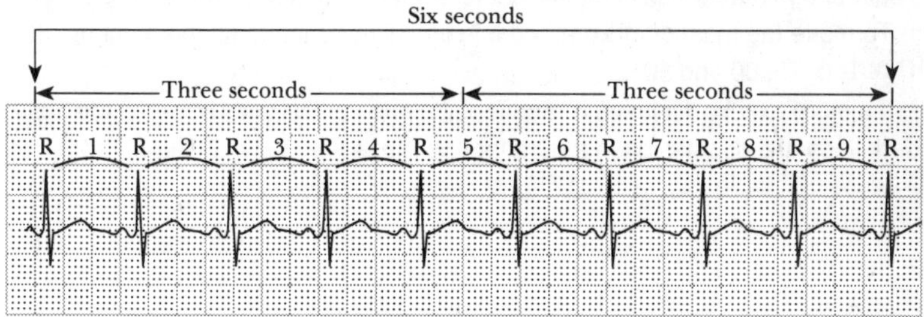

FIGURE 2.19 *Calculating the heart rate by counting the RR cycles. In the above example there are nine RR cycles. Therefore 9× 10 = 90 and the ventricular heart rate is approximately 90 bpm.*

The heavy dark lines

A fourth method to calculate heart rate, described by Dubin (1978, pp 54–64), which is useful if the heart rate exceeds 60 bpm, incorporates the vertical heavy dark lines on the ECG paper. Simply find an R wave which coincides with a heavy dark line and count back the number of heavy dark lines until the next R wave. Each heavy dark line is assigned a number (see Figure 2.20). The first heavy dark line back from the initial R wave equals 300 bpm, the next equals 150, then 100, 75 and 60.

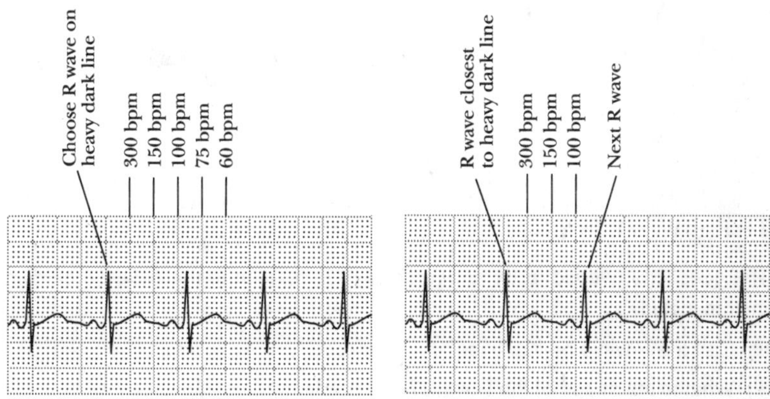

FIGURE 2.20 (left) *Calculating the heart rate using the heavy dark lines*

FIGURE 2.21 (right) *Calculating the heart rate using the heavy dark lines. The ventricular heart rate is approximately 94 bpm.*

Source Adapted from Dubin 1978, pp 58–9

The time between one heavy dark line to the next is equivalent to 0.003 minutes. For example, in Figure 2.21, the seventh R wave is the closest to a vertical heavy dark line. The next R wave is 0.01 minutes away. This is reduced to one 100th of a minute which is equivalent to a heart rate of approximately 100 bpm.

To make the most of this method it is best if you memorise the numbers 300, 150, 100, 75, 60 and 50.

If a more exact calculation is required, the fine vertical lines between the heavy dark lines are also assigned a number and these are shown in Figure 2.22.

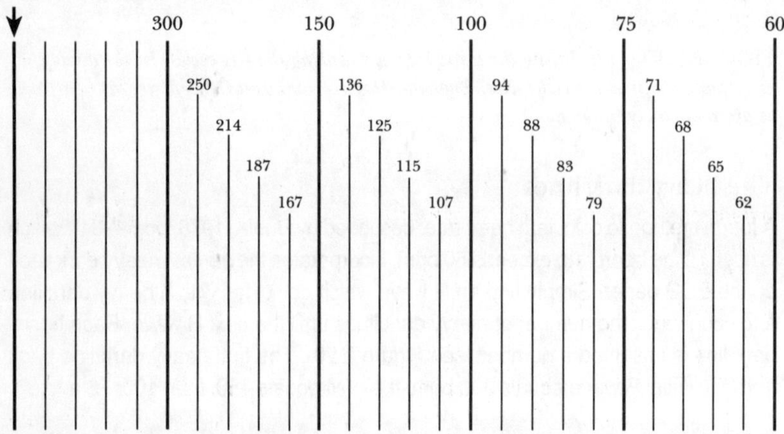

FIGURE 2.22 *Calculating the heart rate using all the vertical lines on the ECG paper*

Source Dubin 1983, p 64

THE P WAVE

The questions needed to be answered here in relation to the patient's cardiac rhythm include:

(i) Can the P wave be identified?

(ii) What is the shape of the P wave?

(iii) What is the P wave's relationship to the QRS complex, that is, does it precede the QRS complex?

(iv) Are all the P waves in the sample strip the same shape and size and are they all present?

This information is important because it tells us where the actual pacemaker site in the heart's conduction system is situated. In normal cardiac rhythm, that is, sinus rhythm, the pacemaker is the SA node and the P wave in this rhythm is rounded, upright and precedes the QRS complex.

If the P wave is absent, this may indicate a rhythm such as junctional rhythm or atrial fibrillation (see Chapter 4 for further discussion on junctional rhythm and atrial fibrillation).

It may be that the P wave appears at regular intervals, but bears no relationship to the QRS complex, as in third degree AV block.

THE PR INTERVAL

The normal PR interval is 0.10–0.20 seconds in duration. To calculate the PR interval, commence at the beginning of the P wave and count all the 1 mm boxes on the horizontal axis up to the beginning of the R wave. If there is a Q wave present, then count to the beginning of that wave. Remember that each 1 mm box is equivalent to 0.04 seconds, therefore the interval length should be between 2.5 and 5 mm.

If the interval length exceeds 5 mm or 0.20 seconds, this may indicate a delay in transmission of the impulse from the SA node to the AV node, as in first degree AV block.

THE QRS COMPLEX

Normally, this complex is well defined and narrow in its width with a time duration of 0.06–0.12 seconds (1.5–3 mm) and should follow the P wave. Under certain conditions, for example when there is a ventricular ectopic beat or a bundle branch block, the QRS complex is broad, and in the case of the ventricular ectopic beat, can be characterised by a larger than normal amplitude and a compensatory pause.

If the Q wave is present, check the depth of the Q wave and note also if there is any notching (small bumps or an 'M' pattern) at the peak of the R wave.

THE ST SEGMENT

Observe whether or not the ST segment is elevated above the baseline or depressed. Normally it forms the isoelectric line.

THE T WAVE

Normally, this wave is upright and rounded and follows the QRS complex and the ST segment. The important aspects to note about this wave concern its shape and, in particular, whether its height exceeds 5 mm or the T wave is depressed.

The QT interval should measure between 0.32 and 0.40 seconds. If it exceeds this duration try to establish the cause. For instance, check whether the patient is prescribed any medication which affects this phase of the action potential curve, for example quinidine or amiodarone.

Once the above information has been collated, you are in a position to interpret the cardiac rhythm. That is, is it sinus rhythm, sinus bradycardia or atrial flutter? In other words, where does the pacemaker site in the heart's conduction system originate?

In the cardiac rhythm in Figure 2.23 the above approach is used.

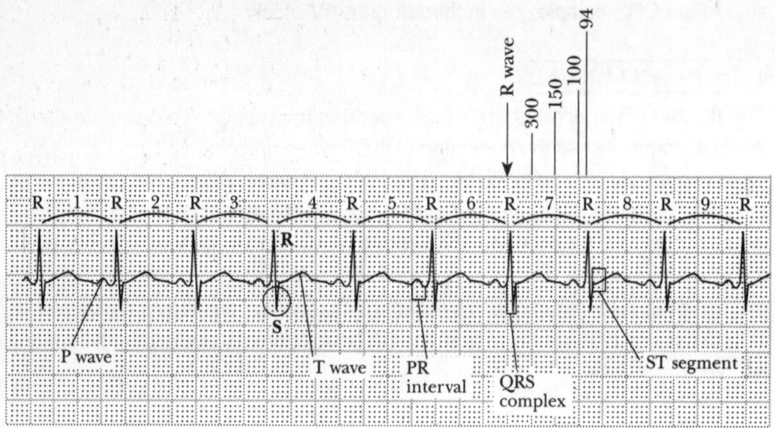

FIGURE 2.23 *Interpreting a cardiac rhythm*

Regularity — Looking at the above rhythm it appears regular. Using the blank paper method and mapping the R waves reveals that the rhythm is not quite regular. There are two waves out by 0.04 seconds, but this is acceptable.

Heart rate — Using the ECG ruler the ventricular heart rate is approximately 91 bpm. Using the number of R waves in six seconds, the ventricular heart rate is approximately 100 bpm. There are nine RR cycles in the six seconds, which gives an approximate ventricular heart rate of 90 bpm. The heavy dark line method (including all the vertical lines) yields a ventricular heart rate of 94 bpm.

P wave — The P wave is upright and rounded and precedes the QRS complex.

PR interval — The PR interval is approximately 0.12 seconds in length and therefore is within the normal range of 0.12 to 0.20 seconds.

Q wave — The Q wave cannot be seen, but the duration of the RS complex is within normal limits, being approximately 0.08 seconds in duration.

ST segment — The ST segment is not isoelectric, but slopes upwards. This may be indicative of myocardial ischaemia, but a 12 lead ECG and the patient's clinical history is needed to verify this condition.

T wave — The T wave is present and it follows the QRS complex. The beginning of the T wave is caught up in the end of the ST segment.

Cardiac rhythm interpretation — As the rhythm is regular, the heart rate is approximately 94 bpm and all the waves, intervals and segments are present and of normal duration, the rhythm is a sinus rhythm.

An important aspect to remember is that although underlying pathology may change the shape of the waves (deep T wave inversion) and the segments (ST elevation or depression), the factors you must take into consideration during the interpretation phase include the site of the initial impulse and the time it takes to travel through the conduction pathway.

Understanding and memorising the normal time durations of the complexes and intervals will help you to reach the correct cardiac rhythm interpretation.

To help consolidate the material covered in this chapter, two practice cardiac rhythm strips appear at the end of Chapter 4 for you to work through. The answers appear in Appendix 1.

In summary, to interpret the cardiac rhythm of a patient, use the following steps.

- What is the heart rate?
- Is the rhythm regular?
- Is there a P wave? What is its shape? Does it precede the QRS complex?
- What is the duration of the PR interval?
- Is there a QRS complex? Does it have a normal shape and time duration? Does it follow the P wave?
- What is the shape of the ST segment?
- Is there a T wave? What is its shape? Does it follow the QRS complex and the ST segment?
- Interpret the cardiac rhythm.

REFERENCES

Boltz, M 1994, 'Nurse's guide to identifying cardiac rhythms', *Nursing 94*, April, Springhouse Corporation, pp 54–8

Dubin, D 1978, *Rapid Interpretation of ECGs*, Cover Publishing Company, Tampa

Dubin, D 1989, *Rapid Interpretation of ECGs*, 4th edn, Cover Publishing Company, Tampa

Holloway, N M 1992, *Nursing the Critically Ill Adult*, 4th edn, Addison-Wesley Publishing Company, Redding

Hunt, D, Carlisle, C, Chan, W & Kertes, P 1982, *Coronary Care Workbook*, Department of Cardiology, The Royal Melbourne Hospital, Melbourne & Boehringer Ingelheim Pty Ltd

Julian, D 1984, *Cardiology*, Balliere Tindall, London

Marriott, H 1988, *Practical Electrocardiography*, 8th edn, Williams and Wilkins, Baltimore

Meltzer, R, Pinneo, R & Kitchell, J R 1982, *Intensive Coronary Care*, 6th edn, Charles Press Publishers, Bowie

Norris, E & Nahas, V 1989, *Electrocardiography. A Study Manual for Nurses*, Cumberland College of Health Sciences, University of Sydney, Sydney

Romanini, J & Daly, J (eds) 1993, *Critical Care Nursing*, Harcourt Brace and Company, Sydney

Rowlands, C 1991, *Clinical Electrocardiography*, J B Lippincott Company, Philadelphia

Sheidt, S 1986, *Clinical Electrocardiography, Cardiovascular Problems in Everyday Practice*, Ciba-Geigy, New Jersey

Smeltzer, S & Bare, B 1992, *Brunner and Suddarth's Textbook of Medical Surgical Nursing*, 7th edn, J B Lippincott Company, Philadelphia

Strawn, R & Stewart, B 1993, *Ready Reference for Critical Care*, Jones and Bartlett, Boston

Underhill, S, Woods, S, Froelicher, E & Halpenny, C 1989, *Cardiac Nursing*, 2nd edn, J B Lippincott Company, Philadelphia

3

TECHNIQUES USED TO RECORD THE CARDIAC RHYTHM

OBJECTIVES

After working through this chapter you should be able to:

- describe the various non-invasive methods used to record the cardiac rhythm
- discuss the invasive methods used to investigate possible arrhythmias
- describe and discuss the care given to patients undergoing these procedures
- identify and discuss the responsibilities of personnel caring for the patient during the monitoring procedure

KEY WORDS

ambulatory monitoring

cardiac monitor

electrophysiological studies

Holter monitor

stress test

telemetry

MONITORING THE HEART'S ELECTRICAL PATTERN

The heart's electrical pattern can be monitored using several approaches which are outlined below.

TELEMETRY

Telemetry monitoring is used with patients who have problems with persistent arrhythmias; patients who have been treated with or who are receiving anti-arrhythmic therapy and require monitoring to evaluate the effectiveness of the medication; patients who have had a myocardial infarction; and patients who have undergone major surgery or who have had a permanent pacemaker inserted. Rather than occupying an acute care bed, these patients can be monitored in a ward near the coronary care unit (CCU) via the telemetry unit.

Electrodes attached to the patient's chest are connected to insulated wires which fit into a cable that slots into a socket in the telemetry unit. The telemetry unit is powered by a 9 V battery. The telemetry unit is about the size of a small transistor radio and can be easily placed inside the patient's pyjama pocket to keep the unit intact. Alternatively, the unit can be secured to the patient's clothing by cotton tape threaded through the plastic loops at the side of the unit. Auxiliary staff at the hospital sometimes sew a small cloth pocket to hold the telemetry unit and this is secured with a long length of cotton tape and hung around the patient's neck.

The ECG signal emitted from the unit is transmitted as radio waves via antennae attached to the ceiling of the ward to the antennae attached to the central cardiac monitor in the CCU. This signal is converted to a waveform (rhythm) which is then displayed on the oscilloscope of the cardiac monitor. If a problem should arise, such as an alteration in the patient's cardiac rhythm, an unclear cardiac trace, or difficulties with the battery (ie loaded incorrectly or 'flat'), these details appear on the screen in the appropriate space of the cardiac monitor in the CCU. Staff should then notify the ward and ask them to check the patients condition and the apparatus. It is important for nurses caring for these patients to have a thorough understanding of this type of monitoring system; to be thoroughly versed in the different types of arrhythmias and current treatment procedures (as set out in the hospital's protocol manual); and be up-to-date in the skill of resuscitation in the event of a cardiac arrest.

If the ward staff notice an alteration in the patient's condition or the patient complains of chest pain, palpitations or dizziness, the CCU can be notified and the staff can immediately assess the patient's cardiac rhythm and advise of any abnormalities. For this reason, it is important to encourage the patient to contact the nursing staff if he or she feels unwell. By the same token, it is important for the staff to keep the patient informed about his or her cardiac rhythm status and whether or not the prescribed medication has been effective.

While caring for patients being monitored by telemetry it is important to notify the staff in the CCU if the patient has to leave the ward for further tests. Once the patient is beyond the sensing range of the antennae, the failure of the link to the CCU receiver results in unnecessary false alarms. Likewise, if the physician decides to suspend monitoring, the CCU should also be notified before the patient's electrodes are removed and the telemetry is switched off.

Patients should be instructed not to have baths or showers with the telemetry unit in situ, not just because of the damage that water will do to the unit, but also because of the expense involved in replacing a single unit.

Each day the electrode sites on the patient's chest should be checked for signs of irritation. If there is irritation, the electrode site should be changed (sometimes the entire lead arrangement may have to be changed). The battery should be replaced every 24 hours to ensure effective signal transmission.

AMBULATORY MONITORING (THE HOLTER MONITOR)

Ambulatory monitoring is a non-invasive form of monitoring and is carried out continuously over a 24-hour period (sometimes longer) while the patient goes about his or her daily activities — either at home or at work. It is used to assess people with known arrhythmias or those who have just developed arrhythmias, for example following a myocardial infarction. Ambulatory monitoring is also used to assess the effectiveness of antiarrhythmic therapy that the patient may be prescribed.

Apart from arrhythmias, patients may also be experiencing syncopal episodes, intermittent light-headedness and chest pain which require further investigation. The Holter monitor may assist with the diagnosis and subsequent therapy.

The electrodes, secured firmly to the patient's chest in order to prevent dislodgement, are connected via lead wires and a cable to the Holter monitor which is about the size of a video cassette. Inside the monitor is a cassette tape, similar to the recorded music variety. The monitor is housed inside a leather case attached to a long belt which is tied around the patient's waist or worn over the shoulder. When wearing a Holter monitor patients should:

- not bathe for 24 hours. If the need arises, a 'bird bath' will suffice
- not remove the electrodes when they go to sleep or be unduly concerned about the 'whirring' noise emitted by the apparatus (which is always worse in the quiet of the night). The tape securing the electrodes can also become extremely uncomfortable, especially in humid conditions, and patients should be encouraged not to remove the tape or tug at the leads or electrodes as this may interfere with the recording and cause what appears to be an arrhythmia
- continue to perform their normal daily activities as much as possible rather than being tempted to sit still just so that they will not damage the unit in

any way. Of course, some of the more physical activities, such as contact sports, may have to be avoided until the test is completed!

- press a small button attached to the monitor if they experience symptoms, which will cause the tape to be marked. When the tape is eventually analysed by the cardiologist, the mark may or may not coincide with an arrhythmia
- keep a 24-hour diary detailing time, activity undertaken and symptom(s) experienced. This diary is to be submitted along with the monitor to the cardiologist so that correlations can be made between the time symptoms were felt against the time the arrhythmias were recorded on the tape (the tape has time intervals marked on it).

CONTINUOUS (BEDSIDE) CARDIAC MONITORING

Continuous (bedside) cardiac monitoring records the patient's heart rhythm continuously while the patient is at rest. Reasons for implementing bedside monitoring include:

- chest pain, which may or may not be of cardiac origin. If associated with unstable angina, during episodes of pain it is possible to see changes in the ST segment, such as depression or elevation
- arrhythmias following an ischaemic event in the heart muscle or those which may be of an intermittent nature and brought on by certain stimuli
- a need to ascertain the effectiveness of pharmacological and electrical interventions, for example cardioversion or the insertion of a transvenous pacemaker
- the management of patients following myocardial infarctions, shock (cardiogenic, hypovolaemic and septic), or any other major insult inflicted on the body's haemodynamics
- the effects of drug overdose, including exposure to pesticides and herbicides
- envenomation from harmful snakes and spiders, for example the Eastern Brown, the Tiger and the Red Belly Black snake and the Sydney funnel-web spider
- use as an adjunct to anaesthesia and as part of the post-operative management in 'at risk' patients and following major surgery, such as coronary artery bypass grafts and the repair of abdominal aortic aneurysms.

Cardiac monitors are box-shaped and can be large or small, depending on the manufacturer's choice and the tasks which the cardiac monitor is to perform. Some units have one channel available so only the cardiac rhythm can be monitored; others are more sophisticated and display the patient's cardiac rhythm, central venous pressure, pulmonary artery pressure and arterial pressure waveforms, with a digital display alongside. Recent developments include arrhythmia and ST segment functions. As well as being able to view these haemodynamic parameters, the information can be stored for a 24-hour period and recalled onto the visual display screen as needed. Data that is not required can be deleted in much the same way as on any other computer.

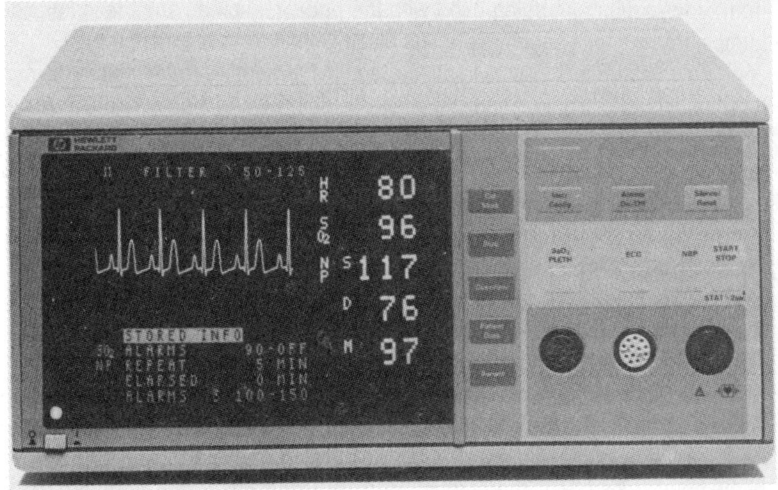

FIGURE 3.1 *Cardiac monitor*

A **visual display screen** (oscilloscope) enables the health care team to observe the patient's rhythm. Some models have a function key labelled 'cascade' which allows the rhythm to be repeated on a lower track 10 seconds later. One advantage of this function is that if there are any abnormal beats observed, these can be stopped on the lower track for an indefinite period by pressing another key labelled 'Freeze', enabling the abnormal beats or rhythm to be identified.

High and low heart rate alarms can be set at the patient's bedside by pressing the appropriate button and adjusting the upper and lower limits according to the ward's policy. Normally, the high rate alarm would be set at 150 bpm and

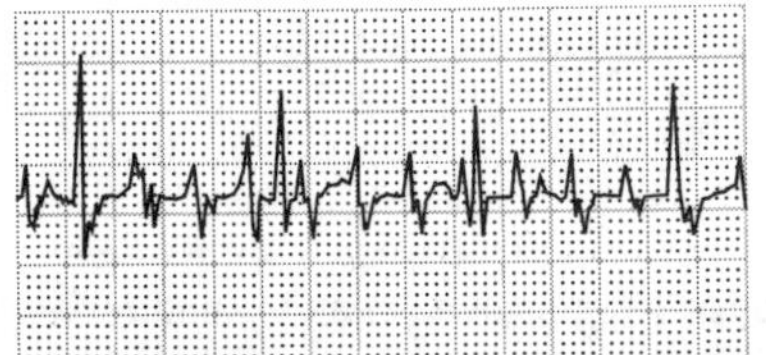

a Interference from patient cleaning their teeth

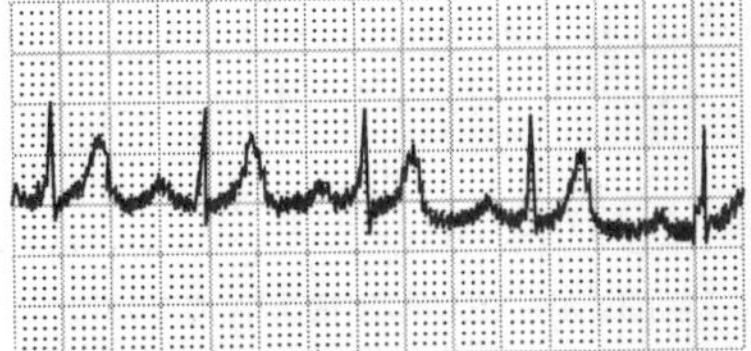

b Leads not connected to electrodes correctly

FIGURE 3.2 *Effects of interference on a patient's cardiac rhythm*

the low rate alarm would be set at 50 bpm. If the patient's heart rate exceeds these limits, the alarm will sound, requiring prompt action by the staff to investigate the cause. Apart from an alteration in the cardiac rhythm, other reasons which cause triggering of the alarm include: electrode or lead dislodgement; excessive patient movement interfering with the trace; and electrical interference from other equipment being used with the patient, such as automatic infusion pumps, transvenous pacemakers and electric shavers (see Figure 3.2).

When an alarm is sensitive to all levels of movement it sounds frequently and this can become quite irritating, especially in a busy ward. As a result, it is sometimes very tempting to cancel the signal at the central monitoring unit located at the main desk without first checking the cause. This is a dangerous practice as it places the patient at risk, especially if the problem is due to an intermittent life-threatening arrhythmia. No matter how annoying the alarm is, **always check the patient's condition**.

The **ECG amplitude setting** is a button or knob used to adjust the height or the amplitude of the cardiac rhythm for better visualisation on the oscilloscope.

The **audible heart rate button** enables the nurse to hear the cardiac rhythm. Each time cardiac depolarisation occurs, a beep will sound. This function is particularly useful where the patient is undergoing invasive procedures, such as the insertion of a pulmonary artery catheter, which have a tendency to irritate the walls of the heart's chambers, thereby precipitating arrhythmias.

The **lead selection button** enables the nurse to select the lead combination to be used for monitoring the patient's heart rhythm (a three-lead or five-lead system is usually used).

Acute care areas (intensive care, accident and emergency, coronary care, etc) select lead II, modified chest lead 1 (MCL 1) or modified chest lead 6 (MCL 6), to monitor the patient's cardiac rhythm. The modified chest leads approximate the precordial (chest) leads in the 12 lead ECG.

There are specific reasons why certain leads are selected over others to record the cardiac rhythm. **Lead II** allows good visualisation of the QRS complex and ensures that the P waves are in an upright position. **MCL 1** provides a better picture of ventricular depolarisation, especially for patients experiencing premature ectopic beats and right or left bundle branch blocks. **MCL 6** allows good visualisation of the cardiac rhythm when there is a tall QRS complex present, as in the case of right bundle branch blocks, and when there are alterations in the shape of the ST segment and the T wave.

LEAD PLACEMENT

Leads are established by placing negative (–), positive (+) and ground (earth) electrodes on the patient's chest. The positive and negative electrodes allow the heart's electrical activity to be measured and recorded. As a rule, the type of lead selected is determined by the placement of the skin electrodes, however, the companies who design cardiac monitors often designate certain colours for particular leads and these may differ from standard textbook descriptions and ward policy. It is better, therefore, to position the electrodes and the leads as the equipment instruction booklet suggests. However, normal electrode placement is as follows.

Lead II

— Right side of the chest just below the clavicle (negative (–) electrode)
— Fourth intercostal space in the left mid-clavicular line (positive (+) electrode)
— Left side of the chest below the clavicle (ground electrode; see Figure 3.3)

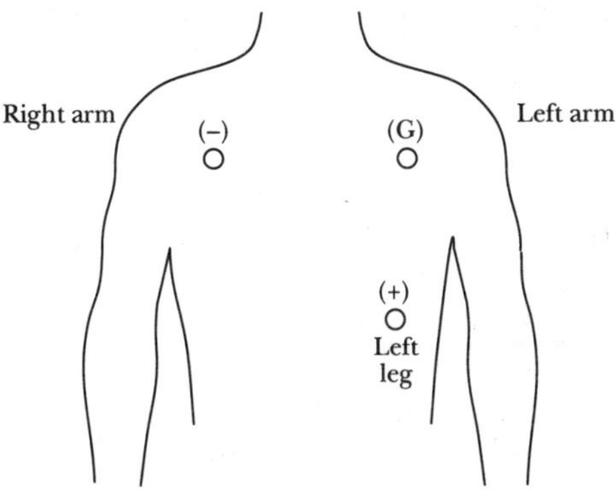

FIGURE 3.3 *Chest electrode placement for lead II*

Modified chest lead 1 (MCL 1)

— Left side of the patient's chest just below the clavicle (negative (–) electrode)
— Fourth intercostal space at the right sternal border (positive (+) electrode)
— Right side of the patient's chest just below the clavicle (ground electrode; see Figure 3.4)

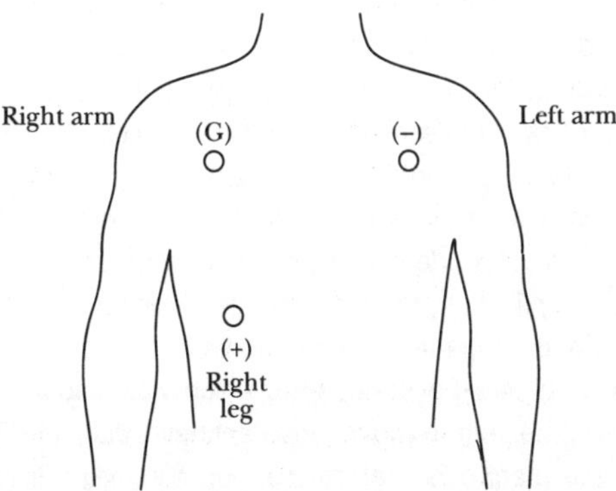

FIGURE 3.4 *Chest electrode placement for MCL 1*

Modified chest lead 6 (MCL 6)

— Just below the clavicle in the left mid-clavicular line (negative (–) electrode)
— Left fifth intercostal space in the mid-clavicular line (positive (+) electrode)
— Just below the right clavicle in the mid-clavicular line (ground electrode; see Figure 3.5)

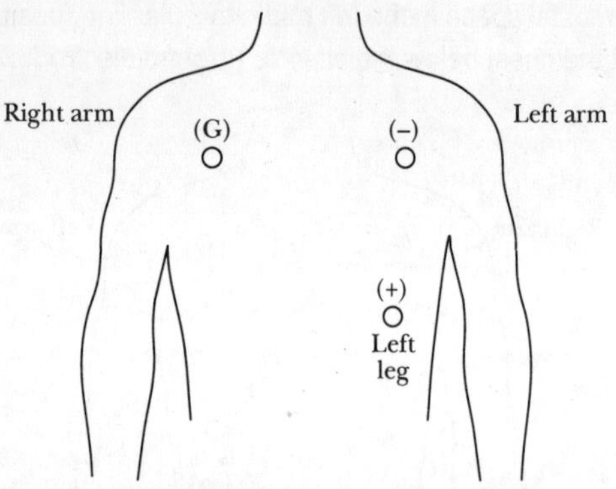

FIGURE 3.5 *Chest electrode placement for MCL 6*

PROCEDURE FOR ATTACHING A PATIENT TO A CARDIAC MONITOR

Before attaching the patient to a cardiac monitor it is important to make sure that the patient and their significant others understand the rationale for this type of monitoring. During your conversation with them, try to find out if they have been given any information from their physician concerning the reasons for being monitored. If not, ensure that the medical officer explains the situation in detail. Extra information can be given in the form of pamphlets and diagrams and by showing the patient and others, as appropriate, the cardiac monitor.

When you are ready to attach the skin electrodes to the patient's chest, ensure privacy by drawing the bedside screens and closing the blinds. Try to ensure that the room is warm. Ask the patient to remove all clothing above their waist. (If a male patient has a hairy chest, to get good skin contact with the electrode, some cardiac units shave the electrode site or trim the chest hair.)

Prior to electrode application, the skin may be cleansed with an alcohol prep swab or another solution nominated by the unit. On the back of the disposable skin electrode is a small patch of sandpaper, which if applied to the skin using a gentle rubbing action, helps to remove loose epithelial cells and ensures better skin contact with the electrode. Before the skin electrode is attached to the patient's skin, check if the patient is sensitive to any particular type of adhesive tape associated with the electrode. There are several types of disposable skin electrodes available. Also ensure that on the undersurface of the skin electrode there is enough electro-gel for the sensing of impulses. If not, replace the electrode.

Next, remove the electrode backing paper and apply the electrode(s) to the patient's chest according to the lead arrangement selected. Attach the lead wires, which are either colour coded or labelled LA (left arm), RA (right arm), LL (left leg), to the skin electrodes. In some cases the attachment from the lead wire to the skin electrode resembles a press-stud and some individuals who are experiencing severe chest pain or who have a slim body build may find the attachment painful. To prevent this discomfort, it is advisable to attach the lead wire to the electrode before placing the electrode on the patient's chest. The lead wires are then inserted into the appropriate position in the head of the patient cable which is then inserted into the socket on the cardiac monitor. Turn the cardiac monitor to the 'on' position, ensuring that there is a clear trace of the patient's cardiac rhythm being displayed on the oscilloscope. (Note: it is important to check the patient's cardiac rhythm and take a sample to place in the patient's medical record.)

The high and low heart rate alarms need to be set at the bedside cardiac monitor according to the unit's policy and a check performed to ensure that they are in working order. The same procedure should be followed with the high and low heart rate alarms at the central monitor located at the main desk because, if the bedside set should fail, the central alarms will be activated if the need should arise.

The electrode sites should be observed each day for signs of irritation, and to ensure that there is good contact between the skin and the electrode and that all connections are secure.

According to the cardiac unit's protocol, samples of the patient's cardiac rhythm need to be recorded at regular intervals and placed in the patient's medical notes. Any alterations in the pattern need to be documented for future management and the appropriate health care staff informed.

EXERCISE ELECTROCARDIOGRAPHY

Exercise ECG or stress testing is a procedure used to diagnose abnormalities of the cardiovascular system, particularly in patients with suspected coronary artery disease. Though a recording from a resting 12 lead ECG may show a normal pattern, when a patient with suspected coronary artery disease exercises, their heart's electrical pattern undergoes changes because the diseased coronary arteries cannot transport sufficient oxygen to the heart's muscle. This is indicated by ST segment depression on the patient's cardiac rhythm.

Apart from assessing the cardiovascular system, the procedure is used to evaluate the effectiveness of preventative heart disease programs, for example, the Healthy Heart Program currently being conducted by Medical Benefits Fund of

Australia (MBF) and to help motivate people to adhere to their exercise programs for their personal well being.

Contraindications to stress testing include people who have suffered a myocardial infarction during the previous three weeks; those experiencing unstable angina, that is, chest pain occurring at rest; and people with severe valvular heart disease, especially aortic stenosis. In this condition the valve leaves have fused as a result of the effects of longstanding rheumatic heart disease or certain types of bacterial infections which affect the heart's valves. As a result, the valve outlet is narrowed. In order to empty its chamber of blood, the left ventricle must increase its force of contraction to eject the blood through the narrowed opening. Sometimes however, the flow of blood is insufficient for the needs of the coronary arteries which arise in the sinus of Valsalva just beyond the aortic valve's outlet. Consequently, the myocardium does not receive enough oxygen and the patient experiences pain in their chest. Undergoing a stress test will not only further compromise their cardiovascular response, but it could also endanger their life. Patients with hypertension at rest and those who suffer from exercise induced arrhythmias may be exempted from the procedure.

APPARATUS USED IN STRESS TESTING

Patients may be tested on a bicycle which consists of a normal bicycle seat, pedals and one pedal powered wheel. The resistance to pedalling can be adjusted.

Alternatively, they may be tested on a treadmill which resembles a shortened version of a moving footpath and reaches speeds of 1–10 km/hr. The slope of the footpath can also be altered to as much as a 22° gradient, with the speed of the footpath increasing as the gradient rises.

STRESS TEST PROCEDURE

Prior to the day of the test, patients and their significant others should receive an adequate explanation by the physician of the test, outlining what the patient may feel and risks associated with this procedure. The patient is then required to sign a consent form, which states that the procedure and risks have been explained in full and that, if the patient requires further treatment during the procedure, the doctor will decide the best course of action.

Patients should be encouraged to have a good sleep on the night before the test and should be advised not to eat or drink within two hours of the test. They should especially avoid consuming alcohol and coffee as these act as stimulants on the cardiovascular system, and patients should also avoid tobacco which has a vaso-constrictive effect on the blood vessels. Patients should be advised not to undertake any strenuous physical activity prior to the test, such as jogging or an advanced aerobics class. Those prescribed cardiac medication may be advised to omit the morning dose until the test is completed.

Clothing for the test should be loose-fitting. Shoes should be flat, rubber soled and comfortable.

A resting 12 lead ECG is recorded before the start of the stress test, together with the blood pressure, pulse and respiration rate.

Between three and 12 leads are applied securely to the patient's chest to continuously monitor the cardiac rhythm. During the test the patient's physical and emotional condition should be continually assessed as well as the blood pressure at various stages or when the patient is distressed.

A doctor or other suitably qualified person should be present throughout the entire procedure and all staff should be up-to-date with resuscitation skills. There should also be an appropriately equipped emergency trolley, carrying the necessary drugs, respiratory equipment (endotracheal tubes, laryngoscope, laerdal bag and mask, etc). A defibrillator should also be available and switched on, ready for immediate use.

On completion of the test, the patient's blood pressure, pulse and respiration rate should be recorded every five minutes until these parameters settle to the pre-test range.

Reasons for stopping the stress test

The stress test may have to be stopped if the patient starts to complain of chest pain which is a sign of myocardial ischaemia, or may develop into arrhythmias, such as increasing ventricular ectopic activity.

Claudication (calf pain) is indicative of peripheral vascular disease and may also become a problem for patients undergoing a stress test.

Acute dyspnoea makes riding a bike or walking at increased speeds more difficult and sometimes dizziness may be experienced which may be indicative of cerebral ischaemia. As well, this symptom may be accompanied by facial pallor or a grey appearance coupled with diaphoresis. All are good reasons for discontinuing a stress test.

Progressive changes in the ST segment involving more than 3 mm of horizontal or downsloping ST segment depression or more than 2 mm of ST segment elevation are reasons for stopping the stress test (Vohra 1983, p 235).

Some exercise laboratories use the heart rate as one of the criteria for discontinuing the procedure. When the patient reaches a predetermined heart rate based on sex and age, the test may be stopped. For some individuals this may be quite acceptable, but inappropriate for others.

Before leaving the exercise laboratory, patients should be advised not to have a hot shower, as this causes the blood vessels to dilate and may precipitate fainting in individuals or compromise the myocardium further in those who have known coronary heart disease. If they must shower, advise a tepid water temperature.

The physician may decide to include a thallium scan with the stress test. In this procedure, the doctor will inject thallium-201 radioisotope via an intravenous cannula before the physical activity has finished. After several minutes, the radioisotope will have reached the heart and the patient is taken to a room where the nuclear medicine scanner is located. A series of pictures are taken which show how efficient the coronary arteries are in supplying blood to the myocardium during exercise.

ELECTROPHYSIOLOGICAL STUDIES

Unlike the previous procedures, an electrophysiological study is an invasive procedure lasting approximately 1½–2 hours (and sometimes as long as four hours) and therefore requires admission to a hospital. It is used to determine whether or not there are any abnormalities in the heart's conduction system. Patients presenting for this procedure normally have one or more known disturbances in their cardiac rhythm. These include the following:

- a persistent tachycardia (supraventricular tachycardia or a ventricular tachycardia) which has developed recently, or may be as a consequence of a myocardial infarction. However, the rhythm may have been present for some time and over the last few weeks or months has become worse
- a bradycardia or a combination of a brady–tachy arrhythmia (sick sinus syndrome)
- syncopal episodes, which may be related to an arrhythmia, and up until now have not been detected using other monitoring equipment, such as the Holter monitor.

The electrophysiological study is used also to evaluate the effectiveness of anti-arrhythmic medication in suppressing an irritable focus. In the study, the abnormal electrical site is artificially activated. If the drug is working in the way that it is designed, then the arrhythmia should not arise.

Some of the abnormal rhythm patterns are due to accessory electrical pathways, which act like a short circuit, intercepting the impulse on its normal conduction pathway and taking it down a quicker route to the ventricles, bypassing the tissue surrounding the AV node, and setting up what is known as a *pre-excitation syndrome.* Accessory pathways enter directly into the ventricular wall or into specialised conduction tissue. The most commonly known accessory pathway which inserts into the ventricle involves the *bundle of Kent* which arises in the atrium (see Figure 3.6) and bypasses the normal conduction pathway, prematurely stimulating the ventricle ahead of a normally conducted impulse. Instead of seeing two QRS complexes on the ECG, the two impulses fuse within the ventricle (hence the term *fusion beat*) resulting in one QRS complex (Underhill et al 1989, pp 389–90). The resultant arrhythmia is known as Wolff-Parkinson-White Syndrome and is characterised by a short PR interval and the presence of a delta wave, which resembles a bump at the base of the R wave. Continued stimulation of this accessory pathway gives rise to a rapid tachycardia, which could place the patient in a life-threatening position.

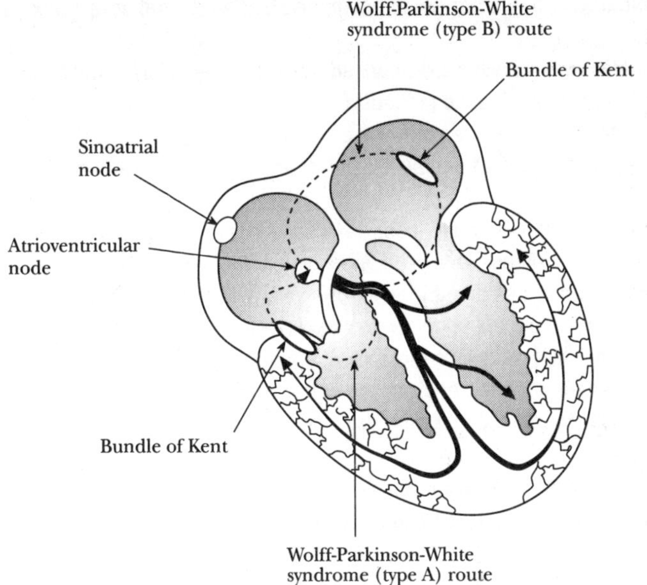

FIGURE 3.6 *The bundle of Kent and the accessory pathways for Wolff-Parkinson-White Syndrome (type A and type B)*

Source Adapted from Knoll 1983, p 116, with permission of Knoll Pharmaceutical Division, Ludwigshafen, Germany

The main aim of the electrophysiological study is to reproduce the abnormal heart rhythm responsible for contributing to the patient's symptoms so that it can be studied in more detail, that is, the type of rhythm, its origins and the precipitating factors. Once all the information has been collected, a decision can be made as to the best method of treatment, which may entail medication, surgery or a combination of both.

Prior to the study the right groin and the left elbow areas are shaved to provide a clean site for the insertion of the catheters. The patient is fasted for at least six hours before the study and once the procedure has been explained to the patient and the significant others (in the case of a child under 16 years) by the doctor, a consent form should be signed and attached to the patient's medical record. In the event that emergency drugs may have to be given to the patient during the study, an intravenous cannula is inserted into the patient's forearm. About one hour before the test, patients may be given a light sedative, such as diazepam (valium) to help allay their anxiety. Once inside the electrophysiology laboratory, the patient is transferred to a procedure table. Straps are placed around the patient's body to prevent him or her from rolling off the table during the procedure. ECG electrodes are applied to his or her chest for monitoring the cardiac rhythm. In case the patient needs to be cardioverted during the test, a metal paddle smeared with electro-gel is positioned under the patient's back (Ross 1984, p 4).

The catheter insertion sites are cleansed with povidone solution and the patient is draped, as this is an aseptic procedure.

Prior to insertion of the electrode catheters, which are 125 cm long and about 2 mm in diameter, a local anaesthetic is injected into the tissue around the blood vessel.

Three electrode catheters are inserted into the heart via the right femoral vein which flows into the inferior vena cava and then into the right atrium. The catheters have a radio-opaque line along their length which allows them to be positioned correctly in the heart under fluoroscopic control (X-ray). One catheter is positioned at the bundle of His, a second in the apex of the right ventricle and the third in the right atrium. If needed, a fourth electrode catheter is inserted via the left brachial vein, which passes into the coronary vein and empties into the right atrium (see Figure 3.7).

The electrode catheters are attached to a specially designed external pacemaker known as a *programmed stimulator*. This device tests the patient's cardiac rhythm by delivering small electrical pulses at a rate faster than the patient's normal heart rate through the electrode catheters in an attempt to stimulate the abnormal rhythm, which can then be studied in more detail. During the study

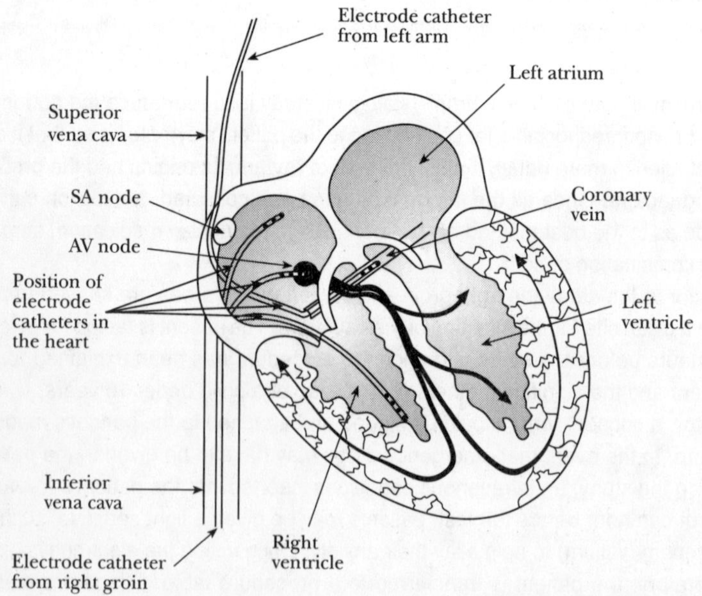

FIGURE 3.7 *Position of the electrode catheters during an electrophysiological study*

Source Adapted from Ross 1984, p 5

patients will feel their hearts beating faster than normal, or they may lose consciousness for a brief period of time from the effects of the arrhythmia. Therefore, it is best to warn them of these sensations before beginning the procedure so that they do not become too anxious (Ross 1984, p 9).

POST-STUDY CARE

On return to the ward, the patient is confined to bed for at least 12–24 hours, depending on the hospital's policy and the patient's condition. The following post-study care procedures are performed.

- Hourly observations of the puncture site(s) are required for signs of bleeding or the formation of haematomas.
- Circulation checks of the affected limbs need to be attended to. Observations include palpation of the distal pulses, particularly the pedal pulses and the popliteal pulses in the leg and the radial pulses and brachial pulses in the left arm. Warmth, colour and sensation of the limbs needs to be documented also.
- Blood pressure and pulse are also recorded at least half hourly for two hours or as set out in the hospital's protocol manual.
- If the patient required emergency defibrillation or cardioversion during the procedure, the patient's chest needs to be checked for signs of blisters or burns to the skin surface from not applying enough electro-gel to the paddle surface or from the paddles being placed incorrectly on the gel pads. The burns should be treated according to hospital policy, but applying a thin smear of silver sulphurdiazine cream is usually sufficient.
- The patient may require continual cardiac monitoring following the procedure using a telemetry unit or a bedside monitor. The rhythm should be checked regularly and samples collected and placed in the patient's file.

Staff should be aware of the different types of arrhythmias which may develop following this procedure and be up-to-date with the unit's policy concerning appropriate treatment.

Complications of the procedure

Electrophysiological studies are not performed without their risks; complications include damage by way of dissection, rupture or perforation to blood vessels and cardiac structures while the electrode catheters are being inserted into or positioned in the heart. An arrhythmia may develop which cannot be terminated by the programmed stimulator. Should the patient become symptomatic from alterations in their haemodynamic status, immediate cardioversion, if indicated, must be performed with the administration of appropriate drug therapy.

REFERENCES

Catalano, J T 1988, 'Lown-Ganong-Levine Syndrome', *Critical Care Nurse*, vol 8, no 5, pp 74–7

Denton, K 1987, *Information for Patients about Electrophysiological Study*, Department of Cardiology, Westmead Hospital and Community Health Services, Sydney

Erickson, S L 1989, 'Wolff-Parkinson-White Syndrome: A review and an update', *Critical Care Nurse*, vol 9, no 5, pp 28–35

Holloway, N M 1992, *Nursing the Critically Ill Adult*, 4th edn, Addison-Wesley Publishing Company, Redding

Hudak, C, Gallo, B & Benz, J 1990, *Critical Care Nursing,* 4th edn, J B Lippincott Company, Philadelphia

Knoll, A G 1983, *Myocardium Vessels Calcium*, Knoll Pharmaceutical Division, Ludwigshafen, Germany

Lossnitzer, K, Pfennigsdorf, G & Brauer, H 1985, *Myocardium Vessels Calcium*, A G Ludwishafen Knoll, Germany

Meltzer, R, Pinneo, R & Kitchell, J R 1983, *Intensive Coronary Care. A Study Manual for Nurses*, 6th edn, Charles Press Publishers, Bowie, Maryland

Norris, E & Nahas V 1989, *Electrocardiography. A Study Manual for Nurses*, Cumberland College of Health Sciences, University of Sydney, Sydney

Romanini, J & Daly, J 1993, *Critical Care Nursing*, Harcourt Brace and Company, Sydney

Ross, D 1984, *Information to Patients undergoing Electrophysiological Study*, Department of Cardiology, Westmead Hospital and Community Health Services, Sydney

Scalzo, T 1992, 'Managing a patient on remote telemetry', *Nursing 92*, vol 22, no 3, pp 57–9

Schweisguth, D 1988, 'Setting up a cardiac monitor without missing a beat', *Nursing 88*, vol 18, no 11, pp 43–8

Underhill, S, Woods, S, Froelicher, E & Halpenny, C 1989, *Cardiac Nursing*, 2nd edn, J B Lippincott Company, Philadelphia

Vohra, J 1983, 'Exercise Testing in Ischaemic Heart Disease', in Hunt, D, Carlisle, C, Chan, W & Kerts, P (eds), *Coronary Care Workbook – A Handbook for Coronary Care Nurses*, 5th edn, Excerpta Medica, Amsterdam

{4}

COMMON ARRHYTHMIAS

OBJECTIVES

After working through this chapter you should be able to:

- describe a normal sinus rhythm
- discuss and describe the common atrial and ventricular arrhythmias
- describe the characteristics of life-threatening arrhythmias
- distinguish the difference between first, second, and third degree AV block
- briefly discuss the interventions for each of the common arrhythmias
- discuss the management of life-threatening arrhythmias
- answer the exercises on rhythm strip interpretation at the end of this chapter

KEY WORDS

atrial ectopic beat
artificial pacemaker
asystole
atrioventricular (AV) block
bradycardia
bundle branch
compensatory pause
fibrillation
flutter
idioventricular
junctional
paroxysmal
supraventricular
tachycardia
ventricular ectopic beat

In this chapter, arrhythmias will be described using actual patients' cardiac rhythm strips collected from various CCUs. The paper speed for each rhythm strip is 25 mm/sec. Next to each arrhythmia is an example of a normal sinus rhythm so that you are able to make a comparison between the normal and the abnormal. Under the heading 'Characteristics', the heart rate and PQRST complex durations described relate to the rhythm strip sample. Drug dosages have been omitted because each institute uses a different protocol.

CRITICAL INCIDENT

Mrs Fletcher was admitted to hospital in the early morning because of repeated episodes of chest pain. She was monitored continuously because, on admission, her 12 lead ECG showed slight ST elevation on the anterior leads. Her vital signs were within the normal range.

At 6.00 pm Mrs Fletcher's husband came to visit and we heard them talking happily. Suddenly, the cardiac monitor alarm sounded and Mr Fletcher called out for a nurse to come immediately. Two of the student nurses accompanied me to Mrs Fletcher's room. Mr Fletcher was standing beside the bed pointing to the cardiac monitor. He was concerned about his wife's cardiac trace which, according to him, had altered since his arrival. One of the student nurses explained to Mr Fletcher that the wavy lines that were visible on the screen were probably caused by Mrs Fletcher moving about in bed. I asked Mrs Fletcher how she was feeling and, apart from noticing that her heart was skipping beats, she said that she felt okay.

One of the student nurses checked Mrs Fletcher's blood pressure. I checked the monitoring electrodes to make sure that skin contact was being maintained and that all the leads were secure. I asked Mrs Fletcher to let one of the student nurses know if she began to feel worse and that they would then contact me. I realised that this was a good opportunity to teach the student nurses how to assess patients' needs and the importance of being able to recognise arrhythmias. (V Nahas' experience)

SINUS RHYTHM

A sinus rhythm is characterised by a series of **PQRST** waves. Each letter represents the electrical discharges or impulses in each of the different areas of the heart starting from the SA node. These impulses occur at regular intervals and have rates that vary between 60 to 100 bpm. Most of the adult population has a normal sinus rhythm. Any deviation from this normal rhythm is classified as an arrhythmia. Figure 4.1 shows the normal pathway of electrical impulses through the heart.This normal pathway is illustrated in the cardiac rhythm opposite (Figure 4.2).

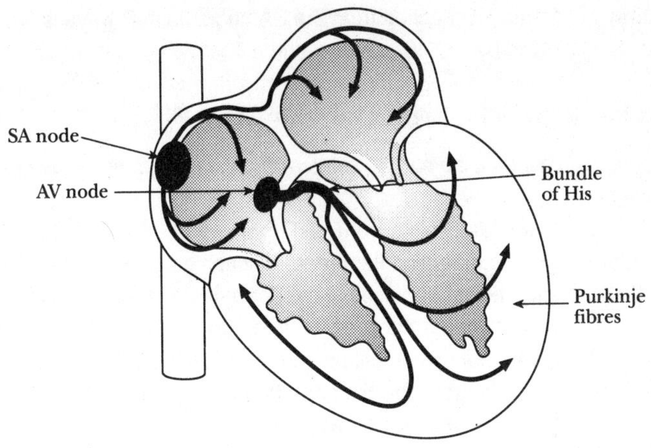

FIGURE 4.1 *Electrical pathway of a normal sinus rhythm*

Source Nursing 1987, p 38. Illustration copyright © 1987 by David E Cook, reproduced with permission.

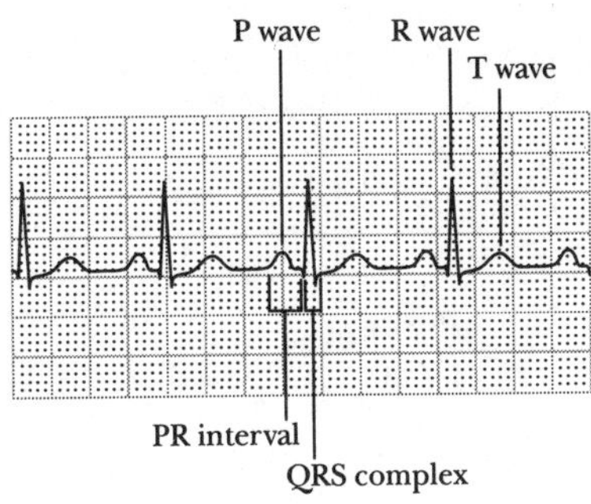

FIGURE 4.2 *Normal sinus rhythm*

Characteristics of a normal sinus rhythm

Rhythm	regular RR intervals and PP intervals
Rate	79 bpm but can vary between 60 and 100 bpm
P wave	present, normal configuration
PR interval	0.16 seconds but can vary between 0.12 and 0.20 seconds
QRS complex	normal, 0.10 seconds (should be less than 0.12 seconds)
ST segment	isoelectric
T wave	normal (symmetric, rounded)

Conduction normal conduction from the SA node; each P wave is followed by a QRS complex and a T wave

ARRHYTHMIAS OF THE SINOATRIAL NODE

sinus bradycardia, sinus tachycardia, sinus arrhythmia, sinus arrest, wandering pacemaker

This group of arrhythmias results from disturbances of impulse formation in the SA node. The SA node retains its normal function as chief pacemaker, but instead of discharging regular impulses at the normal rate, the rate is either less than 60 bpm (sinus bradycardia) or greater than 100 bpm (sinus tachycardia). Sometimes the rhythm is not regular (sinus arrhythmia). In wandering pacemaker, the pacemaker site strays from the SA node to other areas in the atria. When the SA node fails to emit an impulse at the scheduled time, this is referred to as sinus arrest. The arrhythmias do not pose a threat to the patient's wellbeing unless, of course, the heart rate becomes very slow (40 bpm) or very fast (above 120 bpm), and together with the heart's disease, causes the patient to become haemodynamically unstable.

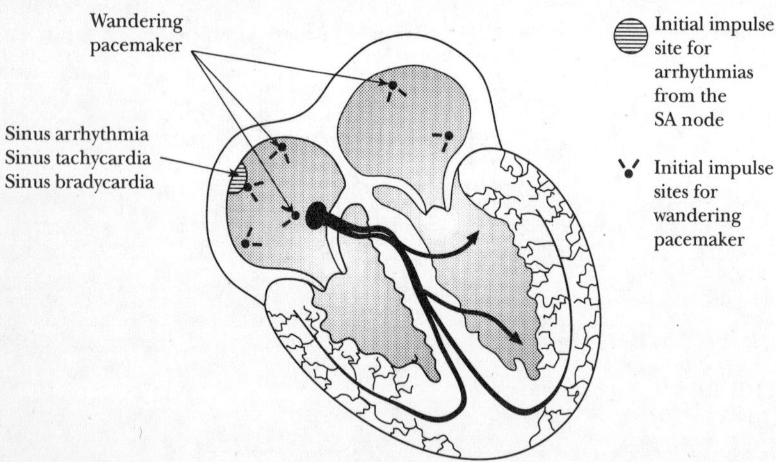

FIGURE 4.3 *Electrical pathway for arrhythmias of the SA node*

SINUS BRADYCARDIA

Sinus bradycardia occurs when the SA node discharges impulses regularly at a rate of less than 60 bpm. It is only the rate that alters — the intervals and complexes remain within normal time duration. For some individuals, such as athletes and fit and healthy people, a heart rate of less than 60 bpm is normal. However, in most situations sinus bradycardia is due to the effects of vagal stimulation, increased intracranial pressure, myocardial infarctions and excess drug ingestion (eg exposure to some pesticides and herbicides). Individuals prescribed certain medications, such as beta blockers (inderal), will present with a sinus bradycardia.

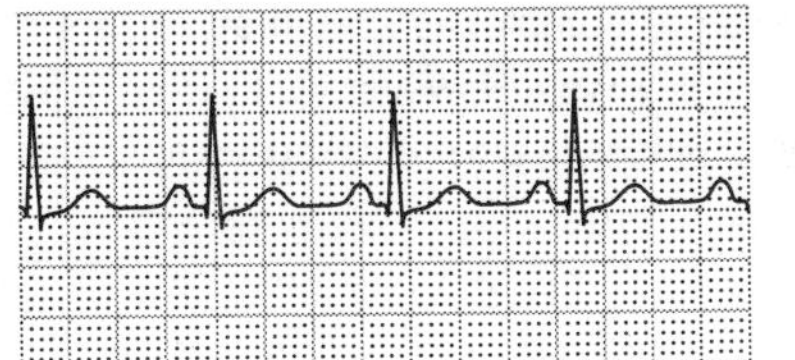

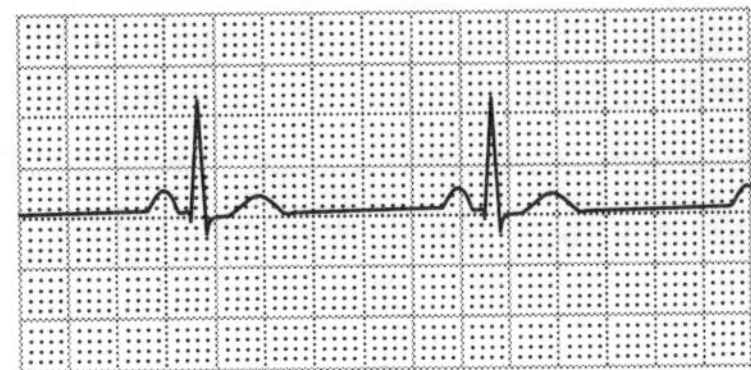

FIGURE 4.4a (left) *Sinus rhythm*
FIGURE 4.4b (right) *Sinus bradycardia*

Characteristics

Rhythm	regular
Rate	normal, less than 55 bpm
P wave	normal (upright, rounded)
PR inverval	normal, 0.16 seconds
QRS complex	normal configuration, 0.06 seconds
ST segment	normal, isoelectric
T wave	normal (upright, rounded)
Conduction	normal electrical pathway

Medical interventions

- If asymptomatic, no treatment is necessary
- If symptomatic, administer atropine, isoprenaline
- Oxygen, 4–6 L/min
- Artificial pacemaker for very low cardiac output may be indicated

Nursing management

- Continue cardiac monitoring
- Document the arrhythmia
- Monitor vital signs for hypotension and signs of reduced cardiac output
- Evaluate neurological status
- Monitor infusion rate of isoprenaline and observe for side effects

SINUS TACHYCARDIA

Sinus tachycardia occurs when the SA node discharges regular impulses in excess of 100 bpm. Sometimes the rate can be as high as 180 bpm. In healthy individuals this rate can occur as part of the normal physiological response during exercise and when strong emotions are experienced, such as anger, anxiety or nervousness. In sinus tachycardia the complexes and intervals are of normal time duration. It is just the rate which changes. However, as the rate of the tachycardia increases, the P waves may be hidden in the end of the T wave, making it difficult to interpret the rhythm.

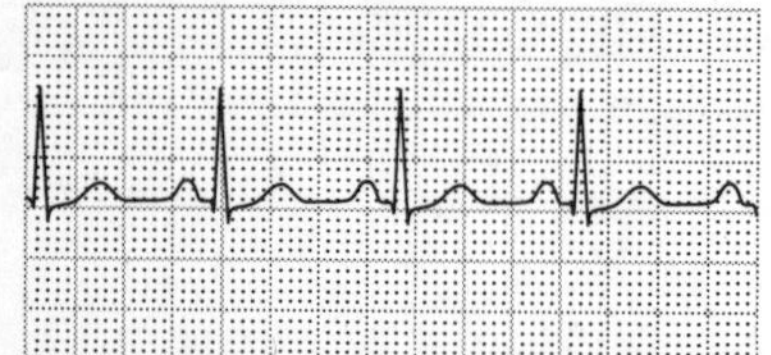

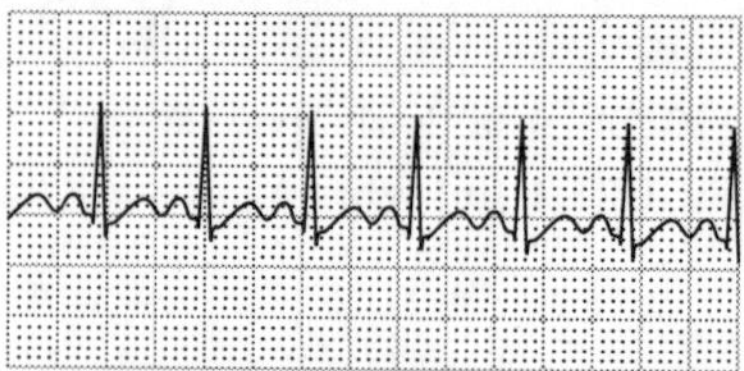

FIGURE 4.5a (left) *Sinus rhythm*
FIGURE 4.5b (right) *Sinus tachycardia*

Characteristics

Rhythm	regular
Rate	136 bpm
P wave	normal (upright, rounded)
PR interval	normal duration, 0.12 seconds
QRS complex	normal configuration, 0.06 seconds in duration
ST segment	normal
T wave	normal (symmetric, rounded)
Conduction	follows normal electrical pathway

Medical interventions

- Treat underlying cause, such as fever, anxiety, hypovolaemia, congestive heart failure
- Cease administration of drugs causing sinus tachycardia, such as vagolytic or sympathetic medications

Nursing management

- Monitor and document the arrhythmia
- Monitor vital signs, observe for hypotension, evidence of low cardiac output in symptomatic patients (ie oliguria, diaphoresis)

- Relaxation techniques can be used as an adjunct to therapy in stressed patients

SINUS ARRHYTHMIA

Sinus arrhythmia, commonly called respiratory rhythm, is due to the effects of the vagus nerve stimulating the SA node. During inspiration venous blood returning to the heart reduces vagal tone, resulting in an increase in heart rate. During expiration, venous blood return decreases and vagal tone increases, causing the heart rate to slow. This pattern can be observed on the monitored cardiac trace during breathing, palpated over the radial pulse or auscultated over the apex of the heart. Other causes of sinus arrhythmia include inferior MI, increased intercranial pressure and digoxin toxicity.

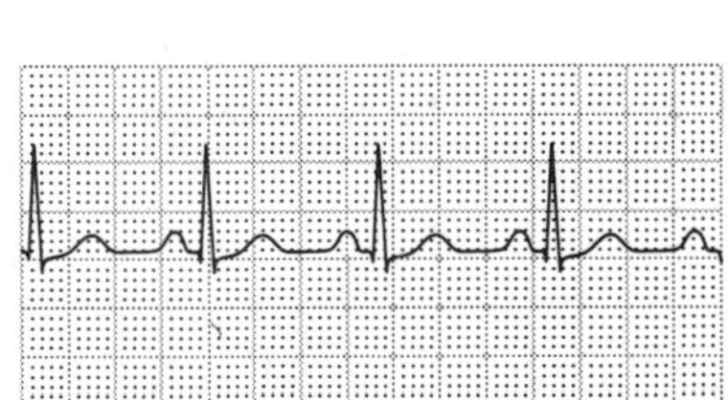

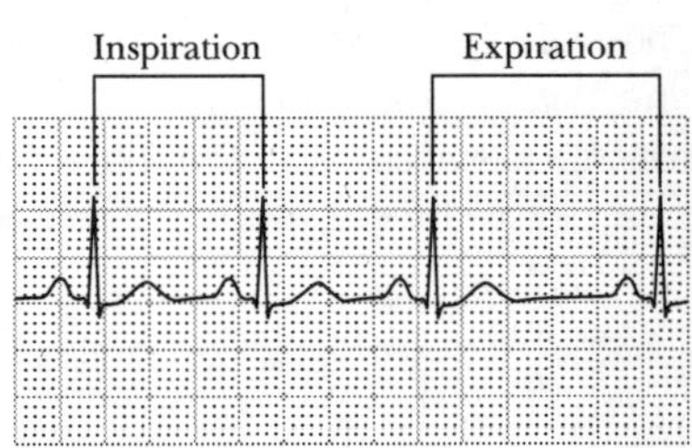

FIGURE 4.6a (left) *Sinus rhythm*
FIGURE 4.6b (right) *Sinus arrhythmia*

Characteristics

Rhythm	Rate increases with inspiration and decreases with expiration (as indicated by arrows)
Rate	varies between 52 and 82 bpm
P wave	upright, pointed
PR interval	0.16 seconds
QRS complex	normal shape and duration, 0.08 seconds
ST segment	normal, isoelectric
T wave	normal, upright
Conduction	P wave is followed by QRS complex and T wave; follows normal conduction pathway

Medical interventions

- None required unless patient becomes haemodynamically unstable
- If symptomatic and heart is less than 40 bpm, atropine should be administered

Nursing management

- None required unless patient becomes symptomatic

SINUS ARREST

During sinus arrest the SA node fails to initiate an impulse at the specific time in the cardiac cycle, resulting in an absence of a PQRST complex for at least one complete cardiac cycle. Sometimes up to three consecutive beats may be dropped if the impulse is blocked at the SA node. The atria and the ventricles will not be stimulated. This is called SA block. According to Armstrong (1985, p 68), sinus arrest can be distinguished from SA block by the length of the PP intervals. If PP intervals are present in sinus arrest, their length varies, whereas in SA block the impulses are discharged regularly (if the basic rhythm is sinus rhythm). However, some of the impulses will not reach the atria or the ventricles. The longer PP intervals will be exact multiples of the basic sinus PP length. Sinus arrest can progress to atrial standstill and so it is essential to determine the patient's tolerance to this arrhythmia. Causes include: inferior MI, increased vagal tone, digoxin toxicity, and effects of calcium channel blocks.

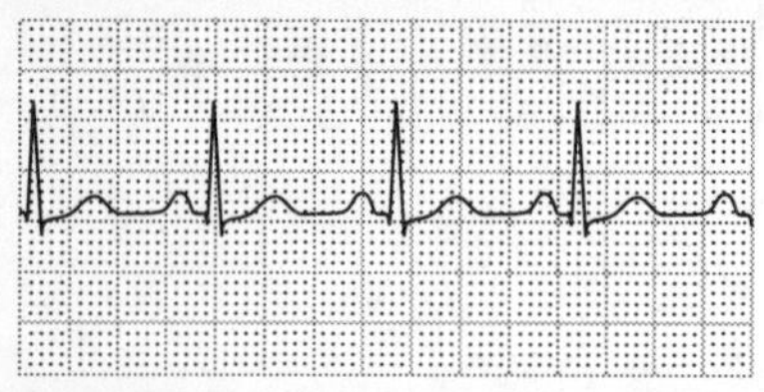

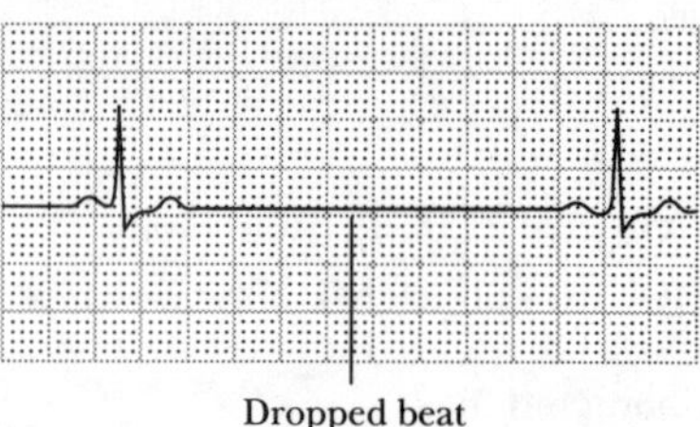

FIGURE 4.7a (left) *Sinus rhythm*

FIGURE 4.7b (right) *Sinus arrest*

Source Noone 1992

Characteristics

Rhythm	normal, disturbed only by a missed beat (indicated by arrow)
Rate	underlying rate, 65 bpm
P wave	normal (missing only in missed beat)
QRS complex	normal shape (missing only in missed beat) and duration, 0.08 seconds
Conduction	follows normal conduction route

Medical interventions

- Treat underlying cause, such as digitalis toxicity or degenerative heart disease

- If the sinus arrest is prolonged, administer atropine IV
- Insertion of artificial pacemaker for recurrent episodes may be indicated
- Oxygen 4–6 L/min

Nursing management

- Monitor and document the arrhythmia
- Review cardiac drug dosage and serum levels
- Watch for signs and symptoms of digoxin toxicity
- Observe for signs and symptoms of reduced cardiac output

WANDERING PACEMAKER

The site of the wandering pacemaker originates from at least three different sites within the cardiac muscles. Its position may shift from the SA node to other irritable foci in the atria and the AV junction. The size and shape of the P wave will vary depending on the site of origin for that particular cycle. For example, an upright P wave originates from the atria and an inverted P wave originates from the junctional tissue surrounding the AV node.

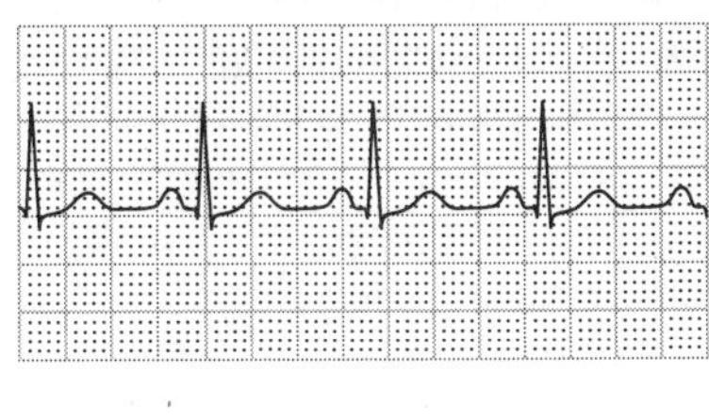

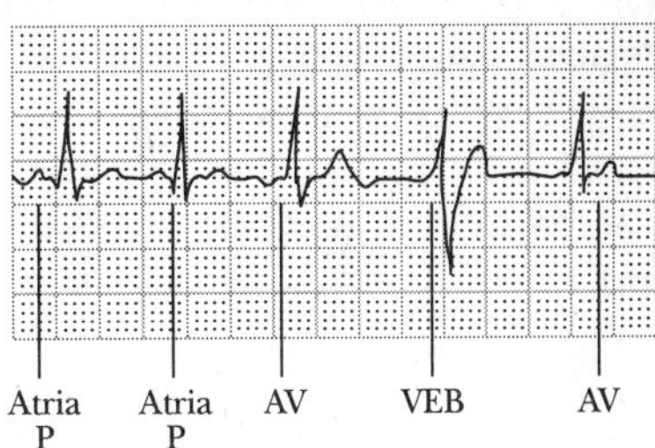

FIGURE 4.8a (left) *Sinus rhythm*
FIGURE 4.8b (right) *Wandering pacemaker*

Characteristics

Rhythm	may vary according to the site of initial impulse; may be regular
Rate	varies from normal to slow rhythm; underlying rate is approximately 75 bpm
P wave	varies in shape and direction
PR interval	may vary depending on point of atrial origin
QRS complex	normal time duration, 0.08 seconds
T wave	normal

Conduction initial impulse varies from one site to the next, depending on which site is irritable; impulse follows normal route after passing through AV junction

Medical interventions

- Treat underlying cause, such as digitalis toxicity, heart disease, or myocardial infarction
- Treat bradycardia if present and if patient is symptomatic, administer atropine IV

Nursing management

- Monitor and document arrhythmia
- Differentiate from atrial ectopic beats
- Monitor vital signs
- Evaluate neurological status
- Use digoxin with caution

ARRHYTHMIAS OF THE ATRIA

atrial ectopic beats, paroxysmal atrial tachycardia, atrial flutter, atrial fibrillation

An atrial arrhythmia originates from an ectopic focus — either a single focus or multiple sites — situated outside the SA node. The SA node emits an impulse, but the ectopic sites within the atrial walls possess a faster rate of automaticity than the SA node. A normal P wave cannot be visualised, particularly in patterns such as atrial fibrillation, atrial flutter and paroxysmal atrial tachycardia.

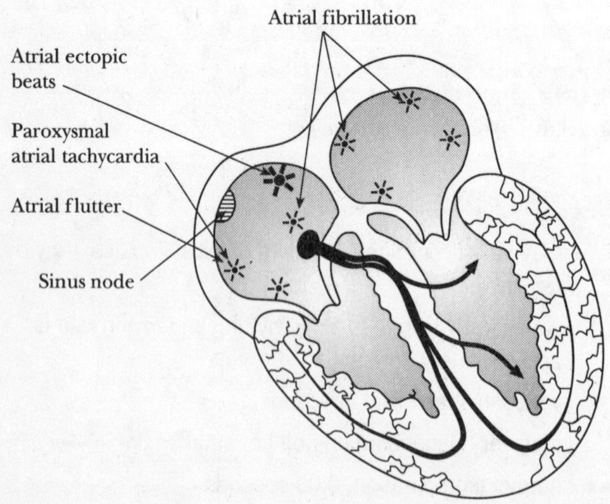

FIGURE 4.9 *The electrical pathway of atrial arrhythmias*

ATRIAL ECTOPIC BEAT

Atrial ectopic beats (also referred to as atrial extrasystoles) occur when an ectopic atrial focus discharges an impulse before the next anticipated sinus node activation. These ectopic 'Ps' often have a bizarre appearance and can be pointed, inverted or notched. An incomplete, compensatory pause follows the atrial ectopic beat.

Atrial ectopic beats occur in 'normal' hearts, but can also be associated with coronary artery disease, valvular disease and inferior MIs, and may also herald the onset of atrial fibrillation and atrial flutter. (Note: atrial ectopic beats are commonly referred to as premature ventricular contractions. The term 'contraction' implies an association with the 'mechanical' events of the heart, whereas we are studying the 'electrical' events of the heart.)

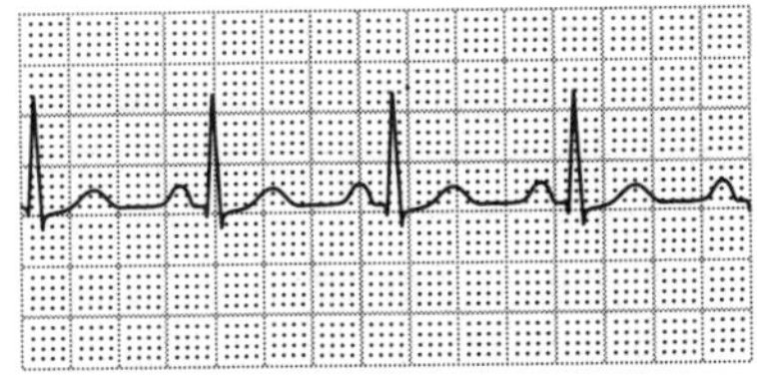

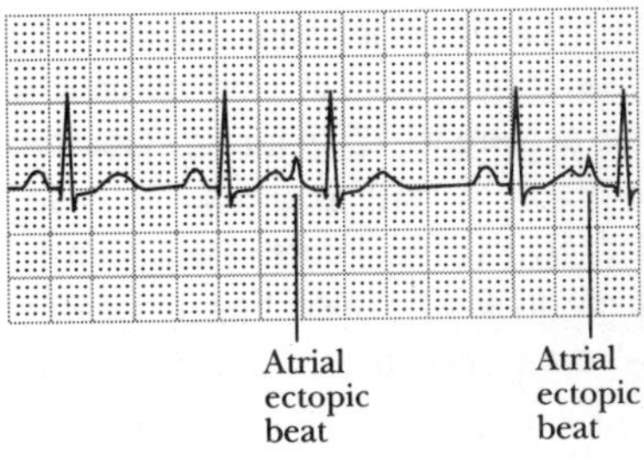

FIGURE 4.10a (left) *Sinus rhythm*
FIGURE 4.10b (right) *Premature atrial ectopic beats*

Characteristics

Rhythm	regular except for the atrial ectopic beats (indicated by arrows)
Rate	normal sinus rhythm except for the atrial ectopic beats
P wave	normal (upright, rounded), pointed in atrial ectopic beats
PR interval	underlying rhythm, 0.16 seconds
QRS complex	normal shape and duration, 0.08 seconds
T wave	normal
Conduction	abnormal beat follows normal conduction pathway after AV junction

Medical interventions

- No treatment is required if asymptomatic or in a normal sinus rhythm
- If symptomatic, treat underlying cause, such as electrolyte imbalance, congestive heart failure, ischaemic heart disease

- If 5–6 atrial ectopic beats occur per minute, consider digoxin. Propranolol or quinidine may be administered

Nursing management

- Monitor and document arrhythmia
- Assess for signs and symptoms of reduced cardiac output
- In the presence of anterior or inferior MI, watch for atrial fibrillation or atrial flutter, as atrial ectopic beats can herald the onset of these arrhythmias

PAROXYSMAL ATRIAL TACHYCARDIA

Paroxysmal atrial tachycardia (PAT) occurs when an ectopic focus in the atrium takes over the role of the SA node as pacemaker. Impulses discharged at a rate of 160–220 bpm. This arrhythmia is also referred to as supraventricular tachycardia because the site of the irritable focus is difficult to locate on an ECG. The arrhythmia can start abruptly and its presence may be precipitated by the occurrence of an atrial ectopic beat. Some patients may experience a short burst of PAT lasting seconds to a few minutes, while others may have episodes lasting several hours. Paroxysmal atrial tachycardia can occur in healthy individuals who describe the sensation as having palpitations. This condition is also associated with people who consume large amounts of strong coffee, tea and alcohol, have mitral valve disease, ischaemic heart disease, or Wolff-Parkinson-White Syndrome. In people with a diseased or damaged heart, PAT can cause heart failure because of the reduced amount of ventricular filling time during diastole.

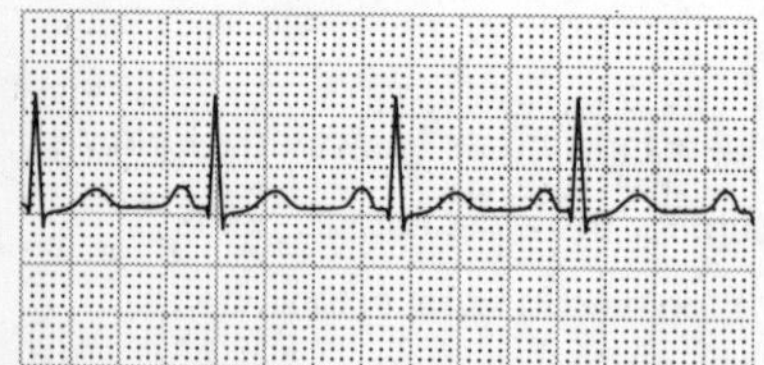

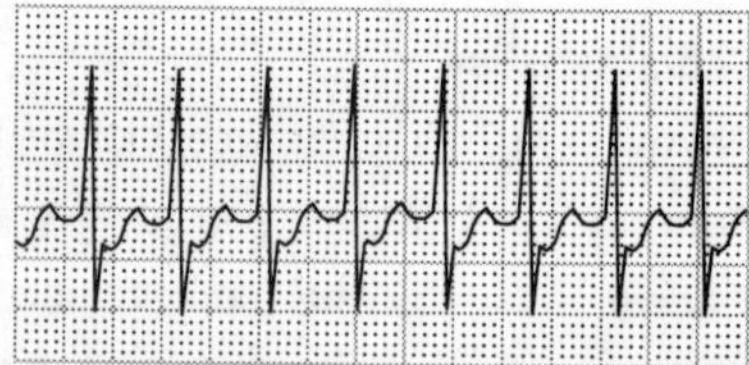

FIGURE 4.11a (left) *Sinus rhythm*
FIGURE 4.11b (right) *Paroxysmal atrial tachycardia*

Characteristics

Rhythm	regular
Rate	167 bpm
P wave	not identifiable because of the fast rate and may be buried in the QRS complex

PR interval not measurable as P wave is not visible

QRS complex normal configuration and duration, 0.08 seconds

T wave normal

Conduction impulse occurs in atrial walls after AV junction and then follows normal route

Medical interventions

- Monitor and document the arrhythmia
- Treat underlying cause such as cardiomyopathy and ischaemic heart disease
- Perform Valsalva manoeuvre or carotid sinus massage
- Administer verapramil or propranolol
- Consider using synchronised cardioversion

Nursing management

- Monitor and document the arrhythmia
- Watch for signs and symptoms of reduced cardiac output, such as hypotension and light headedness, chest pain, shortness of breath
- Watch for signs and symptoms of congestive heart failure
- Health education — decrease intake of caffeine, alcohol and tobacco (arrhythmia may be caused by stimulants)

ATRIAL FLUTTER

Atrial flutter occurs when there is a rapid but regular excitation from an ectopic focus in the atrium at the rate of 300 bpm or more. Instead of P waves, regular saw-tooth F (flutter) waves occur at varying degrees of conduction. Sometimes there may be two F waves to one QRS complex, referred to as a 2:1 block, and

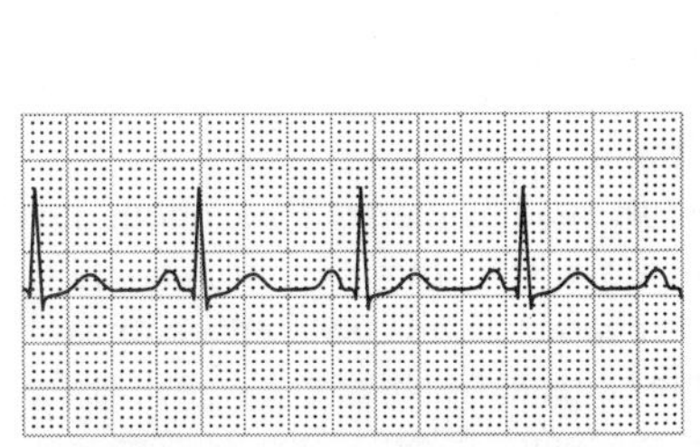

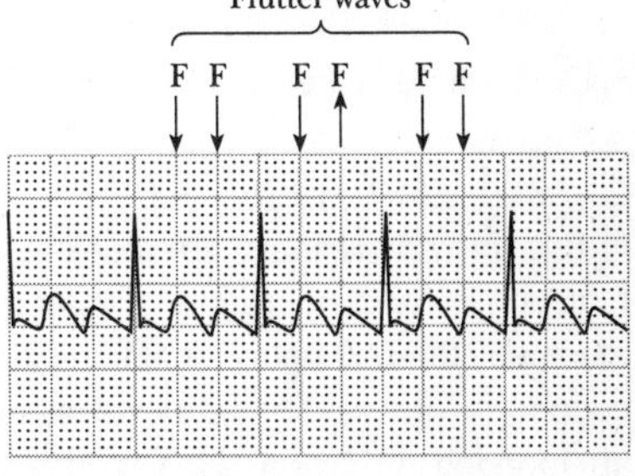

FIGURE 4.12a (left) *Sinus rhythm*
FIGURE 4.12b (right) *Atrial flutter*

other times there may be a 3:1 or 4:1 block. The AV junction acts as a gatekeeper, preventing conduction of some atrial impulses and allowing others to pass, giving rise to the variable block. Causes of atrial flutter include: atrial enlargement, hyperthyroidism, inferior and anterior MIs. Atrial flutter may also develop in healthy individuals.

Characteristics

Rhythm	atrial rhythm is regular, but ventricular rhythm may or may not be regular depending on the conduction ratio (ie. 3:1, 4:1 block). In this rhythm it is 2:1 block
Rate	atrial (300 bpm); ventricular (100 bpm)
P wave	saw-tooth appearance; no true P waves, only flutter or F waves
PR interval	absent
QRS complex	normal shape and duration, 0.08 seconds
T wave	difficult to define
Conduction	ectopic atrial foci, impulse follows normal conduction path after AV junction

Medical interventions

- Treat underlying cause, such as pericarditis, cardiomyopathy, rheumatic heart disease, acute MI, drug toxicity
- Synchronised cardioversion 50–100 joules may be indicated
- Administer verapramil digoxin, procaineamide, flecainide
- Artificial pacemaker may be indicated

Nursing management

- Monitor and document the arrhythmia
- Monitor vital signs
- Assess for signs and symptoms of low cardiac output
- Evaluate neurological status

ATRIAL FIBRILLATION

In this arrhythmia there are multiple ectopic sites scattered across both atria resulting in chaotic, irregular excitation of the atrium. The atrial rate can be as much as 400–500 bpm. Atrial fibrillation is characterised by the appearance of numerous irregular fibrillatory waves on the cardiac rhythm strip, some of which are rounded in shape and to the untrained eye may resemble P waves. The ventricular rhythm is also irregular because of the way in which the atrial impulses are conducted through the AV junction. Atrial fibrillation is associated with patients who have had an inferior or anterior MI and valvular heart disease.

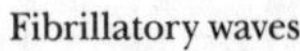

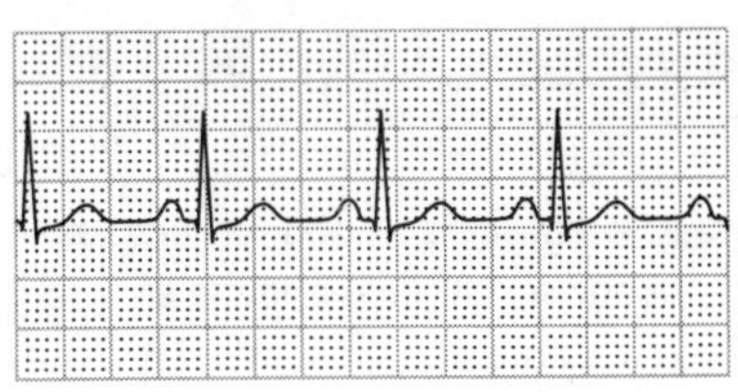

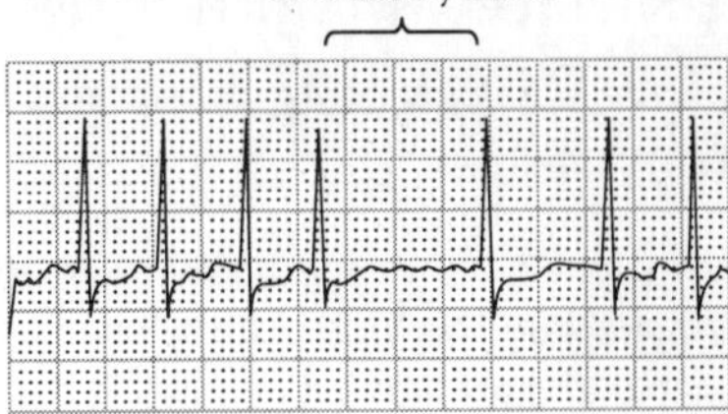

FIGURE 4.13a (left) *Sinus rhythm*
FIGURE 4.13b (right) *Atrial fibrillation*

Characteristics

Rhythm	irregular for both atrial and ventricular beats
Rate	atrial (400–500 bpm); ventricular (varies between 80 and 180 bpm on this strip)
PR interval	absent
QRS complex	normal shape and duration, 0.08 seconds
Conduction	bizarre atrial conduction; normal conduction after AV junction

Medical interventions

- Treat underlying cause, such as ischaemic heart disease, hyperthyroidism, congestive cardiac failure
- Administer verapamil, digoxin, beta blocker or diltiazem
- Synchronised cardioversion 50–100 joules may be indicated
- Artificial pacemaker may be indicated
- Consider anticoagulant therapy

Nursing management

- Monitor and document the arrhythmia
- Monitor vital signs
- Assess for signs and symptoms of reduced cardiac output
- Evaluate neurological status because of risk of thrombus formation in the atria
- Assist in cardioversion and provide appropriate nursing care

JUNCTIONAL ARRHYTHMIAS

junctional ectopic beats, accelerated junctional rhythm, paroxysmal junctional tachycardia

Arrhythmias of the AV node are sometimes referred to as nodal or junctional arrhythmias. This type of arrhythmia occurs when the SA node and the atria are unable to discharge an impulse to depolarise the atria and the ventricles. As a result, an ectopic focus from the junctional tissue surrounding the AV node assumes control at a rate of 40–60 bpm (junctional rhythm). Retrograde conduction of the impulse allows the atria to depolarise, while the same impulse is conducted forwards, resulting in ventricular depolarisation. This explains why the P wave on the ECG complex may be absent, may merge with the QRS complex or appear during the ST segment. When the junctional arrhythmia has a rate of 60–100 bpm, it is called accelerated junctional rhythm (or non-paroxysmal junctional tachycardia). Junctional tachycardia exists when the heart rate exceeds 100 bpm. Causes of junctional arrhythmias include inferior MIs and digoxin toxicity.

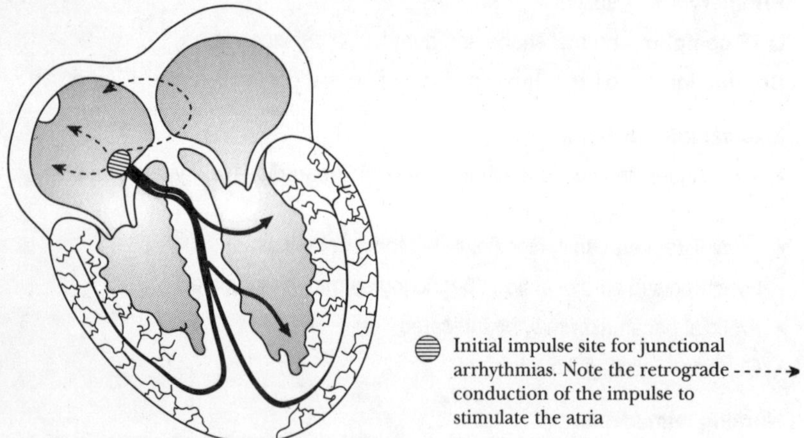

Initial impulse site for junctional arrhythmias. Note the retrograde conduction of the impulse to stimulate the atria

FIGURE 4.14 *Electrical pathway for junctional arrhythmias*

JUNCTIONAL ECTOPIC BEATS

Junctional ectopic beats originate in the junctional tissue surrounding the AV node, taking over the SA node's pacemaker ability when its rate of automaticity and ability to conduct have been affected. The junctional ectopic beat is followed by a compensatory pause to allow for the underlying rhythm to depolarise at its normal rate.

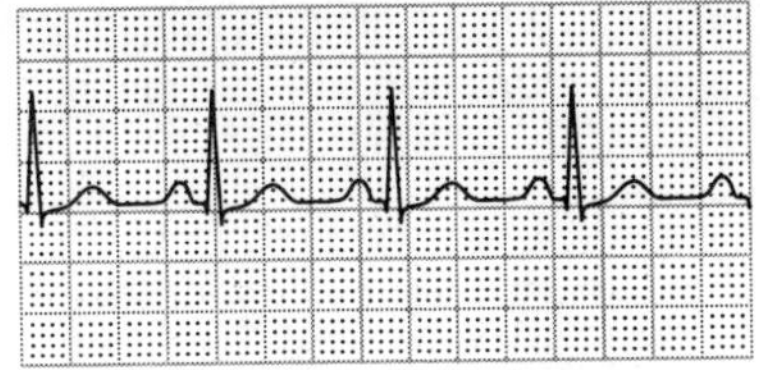

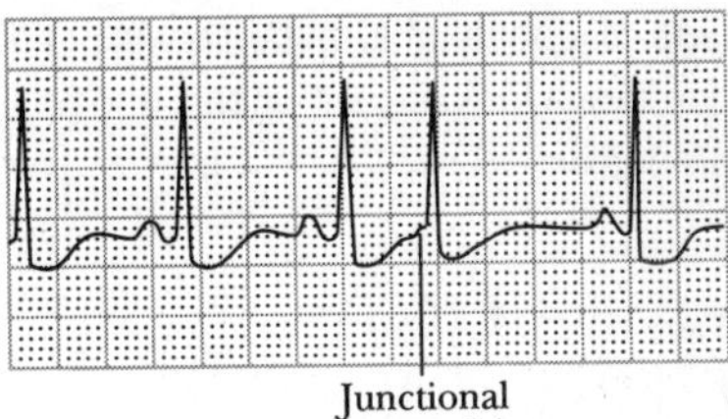

FIGURE 4.15a (left) *Sinus rhythm*

FIGURE 4.15b (right) *Junctional ectopic beats*

Source Hudak et al 1990, p 99

Characteristics

Rhythm	regular except for the premature beats
Rate	normal range for underlying rhythm
P wave	inverted P wave before the QRS complex. In some instances the P wave can be absent as it may be buried in the QRS complex or come after the QRS complex
QRS complex	normal shape and duration, 0.06 seconds
T wave	normal
Conduction	atrial conduction may occur before, after, or simultaneously with ventricular conduction

Medical interventions

- If infrequent and patient is asymptomatic, no treatment is necessary
- If frequent, administer lignocaine
- Discontinue digoxin

Nursing management

- Monitor and document the arrhythmia
- Assess for signs and symptoms of reduced cardiac output if junctional ectopic beats are frequent
- Monitor vital signs
- Advise patient to reduce intake of stimulants, such as nicotine or caffeine as these may cause the ectopic beats

ACCELERATED JUNCTIONAL RHYTHM

The electrical impulse originates from a single site in the AV node at a rate of 60–100 bpm during an accelerated junctional rhythm. This is the most common type of junctional arrhythmia which can develop as a result of acute congestive cardiac failure or cardiogenic shock. This type of arrhythmia can start and end gradually.

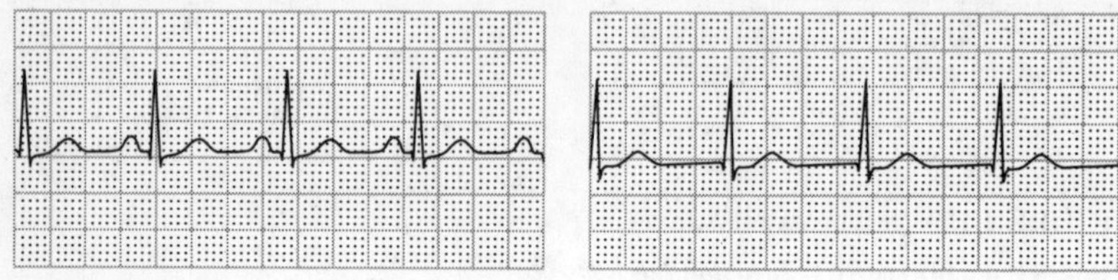

FIGURE 4.16a (left) *Sinus rhythm*
FIGURE 4.16b (right) *Accelerated junctional rhythm*

Characteristics

Rate	80 bpm (usually 60–100 bpm)
Rhythm	regular
P waves	absent
QRS complex	normal configuration and duration, 0.08 seconds
T wave	normal
Conduction	the atria is stimulated by the junctional tissue after activation of the ventricle or with ventricular depolarisation

Medical interventions

- If asymptomatic, no treatment is required
- Treat the underlying heart disease causing the arrhythmia
- If caused by digitalis toxicity, cease the administration of the drug
- If symptomatic, a temporary pacemaker may be inserted

Nursing management

- Monitor and document the arrhythmia
- Administer digitalis cautiously
- Watch for signs and symptoms of heart failure
- Assist in the insertion and postoperative care of temporary pacemaker

PAROXYSMAL JUNCTIONAL TACHYCARDIA

During paroxysmal junctional tachycardia the heart rate is usually 160–240 bpm, but sometimes it can be as low as 110 bpm or more than 240 bpm. The onset and termination of arrhythmia is typically abrupt. It may occur without apparent cause, even among healthy individuals. However, it may be precipitated by electrolyte abnormalities, emotional stress, over exertion and intake or increased intake of stimulants, such as coffee, alcohol and tobacco. Paroxysmal junctional tachycardia is difficult to distinguish from paroxysmal atrial tachycardia and is therefore classified under the heading supraventricular tachycardia (SVT), as the precise location of the origin of the arrhythmia can be difficult to determine on a surface ECG.

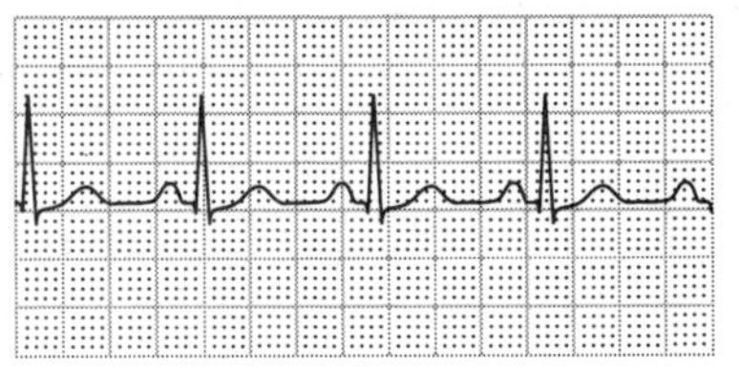

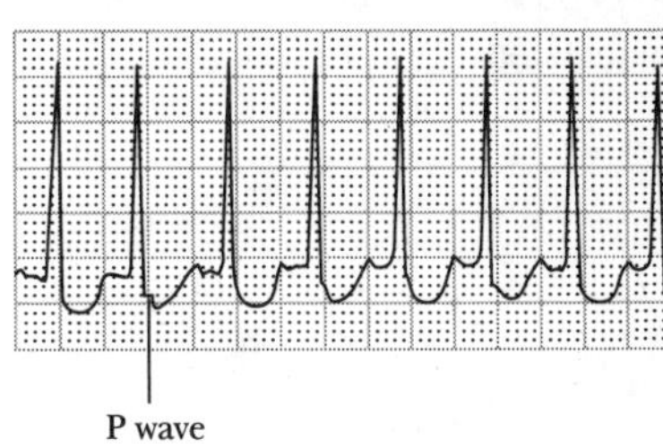

FIGURE 4.17a (left) *Sinus rhythm*
FIGURE 4.17b (right) *Paroxysmal junctional tachycardia*

Characteristics

Rate	187 bpm
Rhythm	regular
P wave	absent, being buried in the QRS complex (a P wave can be seen in the bottom of the S wave in this example)
QRS complex	normal, 0.06 seconds
Conduction	ectopic origin is in the AV junction. However, in most cases, it is difficult to pinpoint the exact location of the origin of the ectopic pacemaker, hence this arrhythmia is classified as an SVT

Medical interventions

- Perform carotid sinus massage while patient is being monitored
- Initiate drug therapy such as digoxin, propranolol, quinidine or verapamil
- For immediate treatment, initiate synchronised cardioversion

Nursing management

- Monitor and document the arrhythmia
- Watch for signs and symptoms of ventricular failure
- Prepare the patient and assist in cardioversion

VENTRICULAR ARRHYTHMIAS

ventricular ectopic beats, ventricular tachycardia, ventricular fibrillation, ventricular standstill (asystole), idioventricular rhythm, accelerated idioventricular rhythm

Ventricular arrhythmias occur as a result of irritability in the myocardium caused by trauma or diseases, such as acute myocardial infarctions, congestive cardiac failure, anomalous electrical pathways and myocarditis. Ventricular arrhythmias may arise from one or multiple foci and are often serious or life-threatening to the individual. Therefore, early recognition and prompt and appropriate intervention is required.

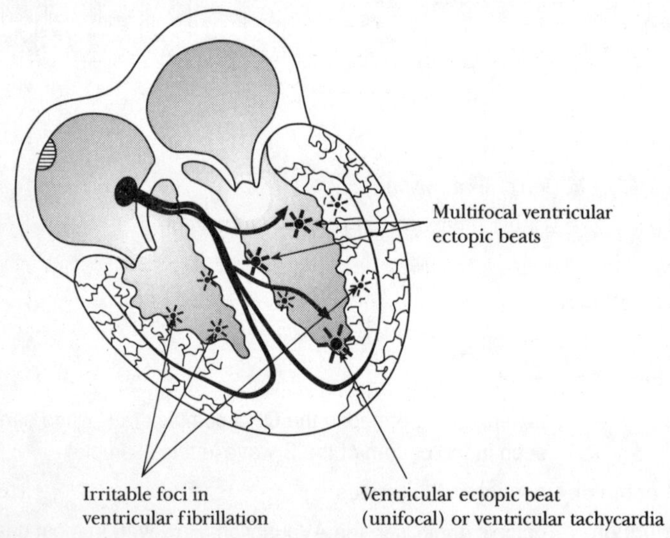

FIGURE 4.18 *Electrical pathways for arrhythmias of the ventricles*

VENTRICULAR ECTOPIC BEATS

Vetricular ectopic beats (commonly, but incorrectly, referred to as premature venticular contractions) result from an ectopic focus (or foci) discharging an impulse ahead of the next anticipated sinus node beat. The ventricular ectopic beat may occur after the T wave, or on top of the T wave, which is dangerous because it may precipitate ventricular fibrillation/tachycardia. It is important to recognise the relationship between the ventricular ectopic beat and the T wave. If ventricular ectopic beats occur in increasing frequency, for instance, occurring greater than one ventricular ectopic beat to seven normal beats, or there are ventricular ectopic beats arising from multiple foci, these patterns must be considered as a warning for impending ventricular tachycardia or ventricular fibrillation. Ventricular irritability is caused by MIs, electrolyte imbalances, for example hyperkalaemia, and ingestion of stimulants, for example tea and coffee.

Characteristics

Rhythm	depends on underlying rhythm. In a regular rhythm the ventricular ectopic beat causes irregularity. Following the ventricular ectopic beat there is a complete compensatory pause, allowing the SA node to regain control as the pacemaker
Rate	depends on underlying rhythm, but ventricular ectopic beats can occur anytime
P wave	depends on underlying rhythm, however in the ectopic beat it is not identifiable or may be hidden in the QRS complex because of the force of the ventricular depolarisation.
PR interval	normal (0.12–0.20 seconds) if the underlying rhythm is sinus
QRS complex	always widened and distorted with no preceding P wave. The QRS complex is greater than 0.12 seconds and can sometimes point in the opposite direction compared with the rest of the normal QRS complexes. The width of the QRS complex provides some indication of the origin of the ventricular ectopic beat. If the QRS complex has a normal appearance and time duration, the focus is situated near the bundle of His; if the QRS complex is greater than 0.12 seconds and has a bizarre appearance, the focus is probably situated in the Pukinje fibres
T wave	usually deflected in the opposite direction of the QRS complex of the VEB
Conduction	the atria may not be depolarised. The ventricles are stimulated directly by their own pacemaker

Medical interventions

- If infrequent and isolated, treatment is not required
- If multiple (more than six ventricular ectopic beats per minute) or multifocal, antiarrhythmic drugs should be administered according to the ward's protocol, for example lignocaine, sotalol or magnesium sulphate

Nursing management

- Monitor the patient's arrhythmia and observe type and frequency of ventricular ectopic beats

- Record vital signs
- If ventricular ectopic beats are frequent in presence of existing heart disease, watch for signs of reduced cardiac output, hypotension, pallor, restlessness, anxiety and oliguria
- Administer medication as ordered
- Reassure the patient and provide emotional support

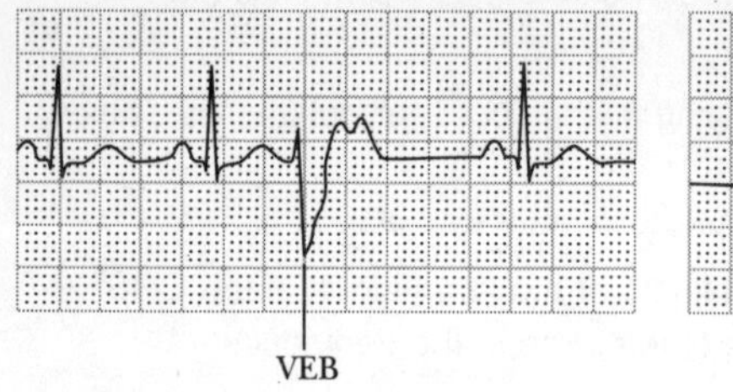

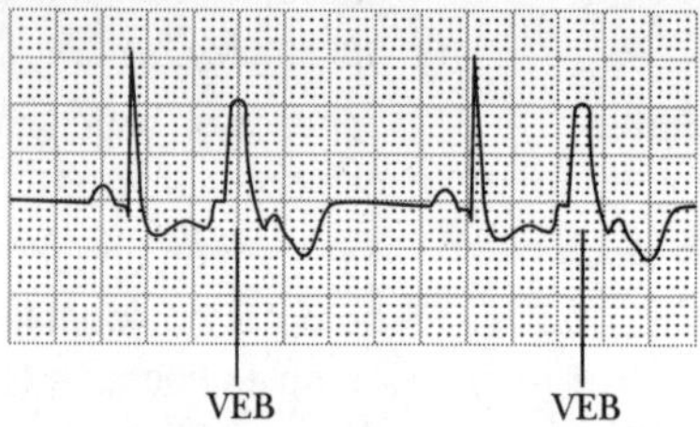

FIGURE 4.19a (left) *Unifocal ventricular ectopic beats (all have the same shape because they arise from the same focus)*

FIGURE 4.19b (right) *Ventricular bigeminy (one normal beat followed by an ectopic beat)*

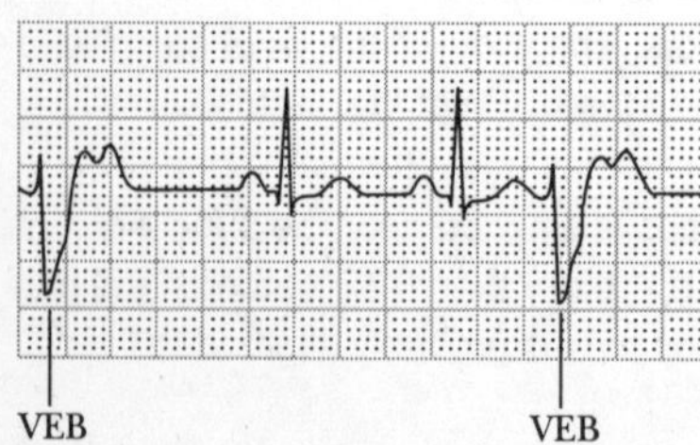

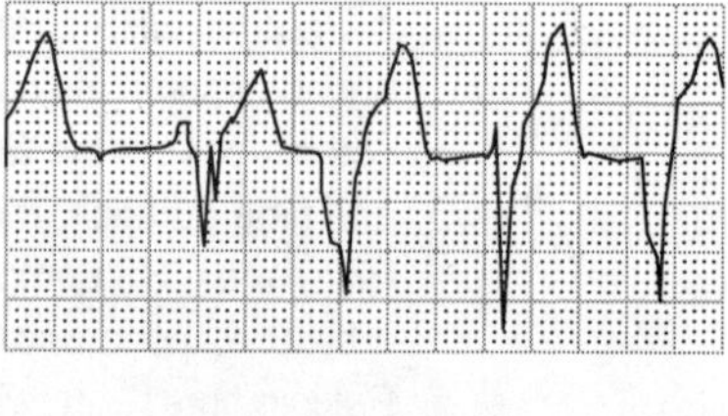

FIGURE 4.19c (left) *Ventricular trigeminy (two normal beats followed by a ventricular ectopic beat)*

FIGURE 4.19d (right) *Sequential ventricular ectopic beats (occur in twos or threes)*

VENTRICULAR TACHYCARDIA

Ventricular tachycardia develops when there are three or more consecutive ventricular ectopic beats and the heart rate exceeds 100 bpm. Such activity is due to enhanced automaticity and re-entry within the Purkinje fibres. Even though the ventricular rate may be as much as 200 bpm, the atrial rate cannot be measured because the P waves are not visible, but hidden in the QRS complex. Two other forms of ventricular tachycardia exist and it is important for you to be able to distinguish one form from the other.

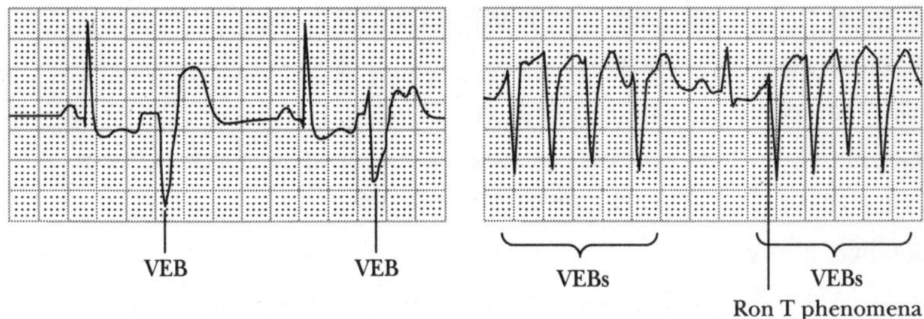

FIGURE 4.19e (left) *Multifocal ventricular ectopic beats (originate from different ventricular foci, so appearance varies)*

FIGURE 4.19f (right) *R on T pattern VEBs (strike the T wave of the preceding QRS complex, precipitating ventricular fibrillation). The R wave of the ventricular beat occurs at the peak or on the top of the T wave. This is the most vulnerable point in the cardiac cycle where the specialised cardiac cells are capable of conducting another impulse. The rhythm that results is ventricular tachycardia (sometimes fibrillation) and is life-threatening.*

Torsades de Pointes — the ventricular rate is 150–250 bpm and the QRS complex is wide and rotates about the baseline, hence the phrase 'dancing' or 'twisting' on the points.

R on T phenomena — the R wave of a ventricular ectopic beat coincides with the peak of the T wave of the previous beat. As repolarisation is incomplete, the cells are capable of receiving further stimulation, which results in a rhythm such as ventricular tachycardia or ventricular fibrillation.

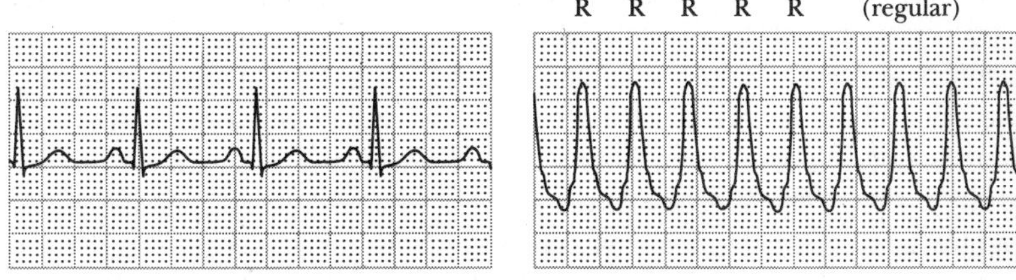

FIGURE 4.20a (left) *Sinus rhythm*

FIGURE 4.20b (right) *Ventricular tachycardia*

Causes of ventricular tachycardia include: MIs, hypokalaemia, cardiomyopathy, digoxin toxicity and quinidine. Ventricular tachycardia is a life-threatening arrhythmia which requires immediate recognition and prompt intervention.

Characteristics

Rhythm regular

Rate ventricular (180 bpm), but can range from 100 to 200 bpm

P wave not present, or hidden in QRS complex

PR interval not present

QRS complex uniform configuration

Conduction the ventricles are directly stimulated by an ectopic focus within the Purkinje fibre network

Medical interventions

- Treat underlying cause, such as ischaemic heart disease, aneurysm, rheumatic heart disease, metabolic disturbances and cardiomyopathy
- If unconscious, defibrillate and continue CPR
- If conscious, administer lignocaine procainamide, bretylium tosylate or magnesium sulphate

Nursing management

- Monitor and document the arrhythmia
- Monitor vital signs
- Assess level of consciousness as some patients become unresponsive with onset of arrhythmia
- Watch for signs and symptoms of reduced cardiac output, for example confusion, hypotension or syncope
- Assist in CPR

VENTRICULAR FIBRILLATION

Ventricular fibrillation is a lethal arrhythmia and is characterised by chaotic, uncoordinated ventricular depolarisation. It is usually initiated by the R wave of a ventricular ectopic beat striking the peak of the T wave in the preceding beat. Because of the chaotic electrical activity, the muscle mass just quivers and cardiac output falls rapidly, rendering the individual unconscious with the risk of death ensuing. Therefore, prompt recognition of the warning signs, such as frequent ventricular ectopic beats or the relationship of these to the T waves (R on T), may prevent this arrhythmia from occurring. Other causes of ventricular fibrillation include: MIs, hypokalaemia, hypothermia, severe acidosis and alkalosis.

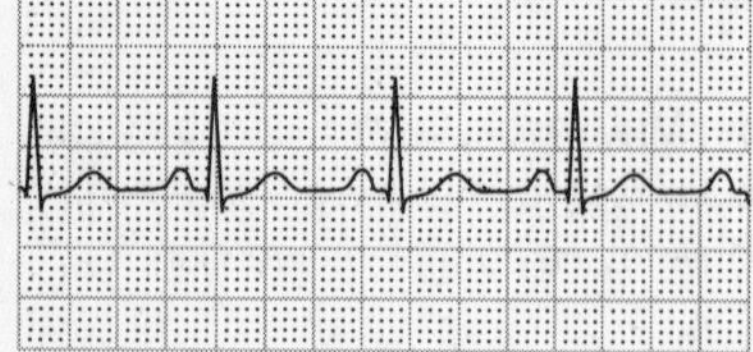

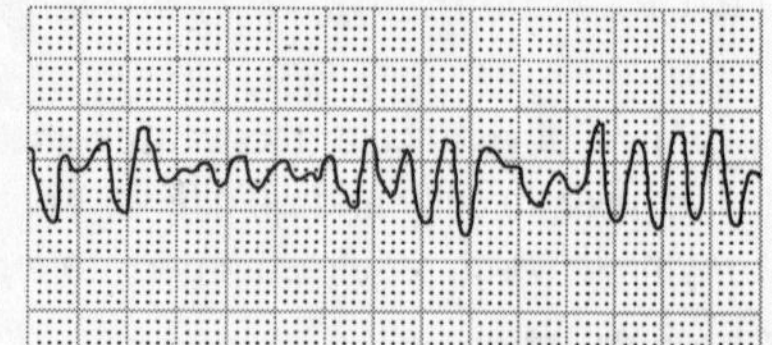

FIGURE 4.21a (left) *Sinus rhythm*

FIGURE 4.21b (right) *Ventricular fibrillation*

Characteristics

Rhythm	irregular, chaotic
Rate	cannot be determined
P wave	absent
PR interval	absent
QRS complex	replaced by f waves
Conduction	uncoordinated ventricular depolarisation

Medical interventions

- Defibrillate if ventricular fibrillation is coarse; if ventricular fibrillation is fine (looks like a wavy line), give adrenaline and commence CPR. (For more information, the Australian Resuscitation Council provides guidelines for advanced life support. These guidelines appear in Figure 5.6 on p 112.)

Nursing management

- Identify the arrhythmia and act according to the ward protocol
- Monitor and document the arrhythmia
- Monitor vital signs
- Assist in CPR

VENTRICULAR STANDSTILL

In ventricular standstill (also called ventricular asystole, cardiac standstill and cardiac arrest) the electrical impulse from the SA node doesn't reach the ventricles. P waves are present on the cardiac trace, but the QRS complex and T waves are absent. If this arrhythmia is allowed to progress, an ectopic pacemaker in the Purkinje fibres takes over as pacemaker and widened QRS complexes will appear. There will be no P waves and the heart rate will be 20 bpm or less. Ventricular standstill is usually associated with third degree AV block, or follows acute MI, acute respiratory failure, ischaemic heart disease or cardiogenic shock.

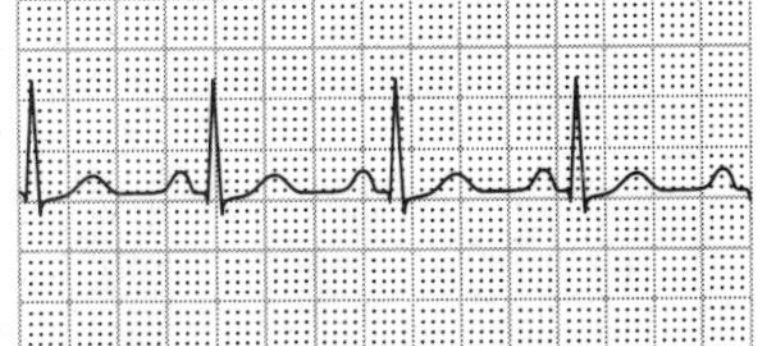

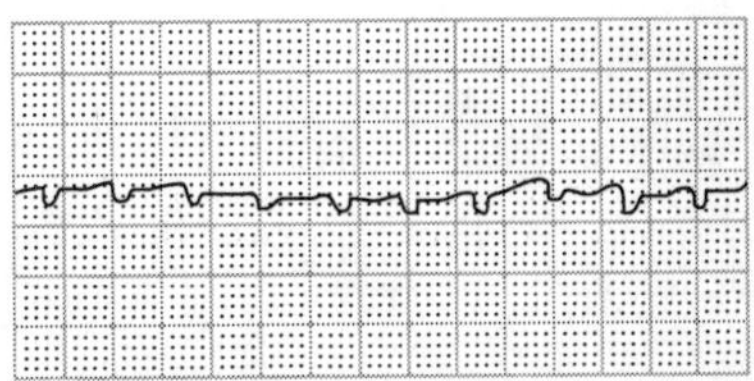

FIGURE 4.22a (left) *Sinus rhythm*

FIGURE 4.22b (right) *Ventricular standstill*

The individual is rendered unconscious (no cardiac output is present) and unless resuscitated, death ensues.

Characteristics

Rhythm	no ventricular activity; atrial activity dependent on origin of impulse
Rate	atrial regular, but dependent on origin of impulse; no ventricular depolarisation
P wave	present
PR interval	absent
QRS complex	absent
Conduction	no conduction through the ventricles

Medical interventions

- Commence CPR and defibrillation when required
- Transvenous pacemaker may be indicated
- Advanced life support
- Treat underlying cause, such as MI, cardiorespiratory arrest

Nursing management

- Confirm asystole and commence CPR
- Document the arrhythmia
- Document signs, such as apnoea, no palpable pulse, loss of consciousness and no blood pressure
- Assist in CPR

IDIOVENTRICULAR RHYTHM

Idioventricular rhythm (often referred to as ventricular escape rhythm) arises when all other supraventricular pacemakers (SA node, AV junction, bundle of His,

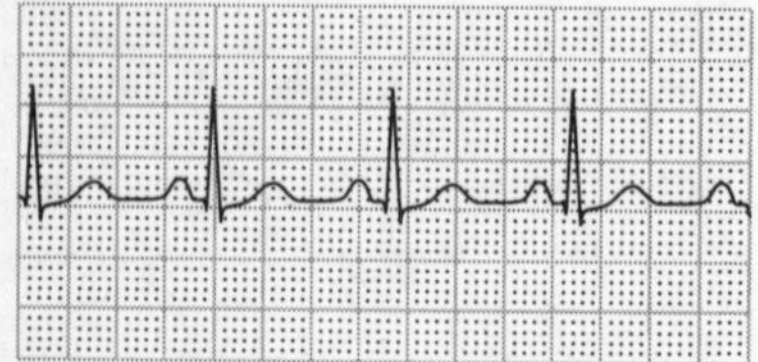

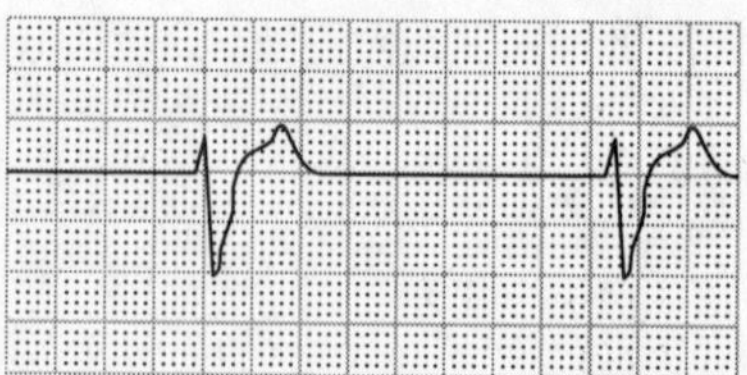

FIGURE 4.23a (left) *Sinus rhythm*

FIGURE 4.23b (right) *Idioventricular rhythm*

bundle branches) fail to elicit an electrical impulse. The ventricles take over as pacemaker, firing at their own inherent rate of 30–40 bpm.

Characteristics

Rate	35 bpm (ventricles usually 30–40 bpm);
Rhythm	regular RR intervals
P wave	absent, but sometimes there is retrograde conduction through the AV node and a wave may occur after the QRS complex (seen in the ST segment as a notch)
QRS complex	wide (0.20 seconds) and bizarre
Conduction	electrical discharge arises from the Purkinje fibres or ventricular myocardium

Medical interventions

- Immediate cardiopulmonary resuscitation is required to reverse the consequences of reduced cardiac output
- Administer 100% oxygen
- Administer adrenaline
- Administer atropine
- A temporary pacemaker may be indicated to improve cardiac output

Nursing management

- Assist in cardiopulmonary resuscitation
- Monitor and document the arrhythmia
- Monitor vital signs
- Document signs of reduced cardiac output, such as hypotension, syncope and shock
- Assist in the insertion of pacemaker when indicated

ACCELERATED IDIOVENTRICULAR RHYTHM

Accelerated idioventricular rhythm is often described as 'slow VT' because the beats are similar in configuration to ventricular ectopic beats. Although the arrhythmia originates from low down in the ventricular pathway and should possess a heart rate of 20–40 bpm, it actually has a faster rate of 50–100 bpm, hence the title 'accelerated'.

This arrhythmia occurs when the SA node fails as the heart's pacemaker and the ventricular pacemaker takes over. However, when the SA node recovers, the ectopic focus retreats. Causes of accelerated ventricular rhythm include MI and digoxin toxicity.

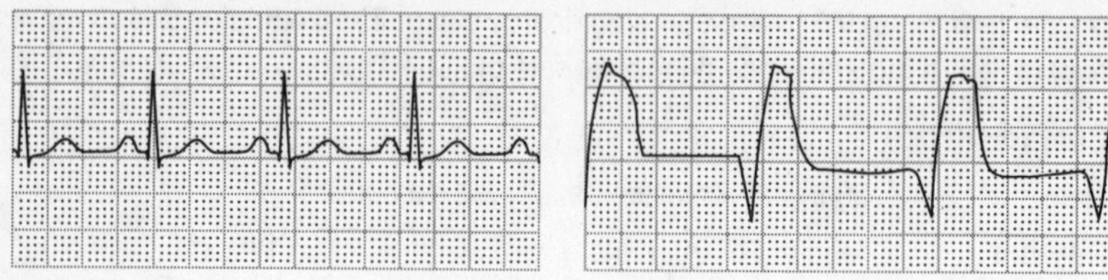

FIGURE 4.24a (left) *Sinus rhythm*
FIGURE 4.24b (right) *Accelerated idioventricular rhythm*

Characteristics

Rate	60 bpm (usually 50–100 bpm)
Rhythm	regular RR intervals; resembles 'slow VT'
P wave	absent (normally hidden in QRS complex)
QRS complex	wide (greater than 0.12 seconds) and bizarre
T wave	caught up in ST segment
Conduction	pacemaker site is in the bundle branches, Purkinje fibres or myocardium

Medical interventions

- Treat the underlying cause of the arrhythmia
- The arrhythmia is self-limiting and may return to sinus rhythm
- If the episode is prolonged, treat the patient as for ventricular tachycardia

Nursing management

- Monitor and document the arrhythmia
- Document signs and symptoms of hypotension and shock
- Monitor vital signs

ATRIOVENTRICULAR BLOCKS (CONDUCTION DISORDERS)

first degree AV block, second degree AV block, third degree AV block

Atrioventricular blocks occur when impulses originating in the SA node are delayed at the AV node or the tissue surrounding it for (1) a uniform time (first degree AV block); (2) a gradually lengthening time (second degree AV block); or (3) the impulse is blocked completely (third degree AV block). Conditions which give rise to conduction disorders include degenerative heart disease, primarily involving the blood vessels and particularly those supplying nutrients to the SA node and the AV node. The effects of trauma or damage to the heart as in acute MIs also lead to conduction disorders. In caring for patients who present with any one or a combination of these conditions, nurses must be on the lookout for the development of any of the conduction disorders so that appropriate interventions can be instituted.

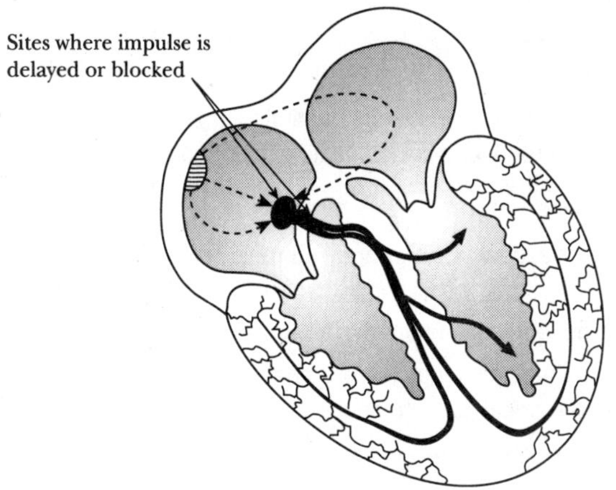

FIGURE 4.25 *Electrical pathway for AV blocks (conduction disorders)*

FIRST DEGREE AV HEART BLOCK

First degree AV blocks occur when there is a delay in the transmission of impulses through the AV node (or junctional tissue) to the ventricles. This rhythm is characterised by a long PR interval greater than 0.20 seconds, due to the interruption in the conduction system. This arrhythmia is commonly associated with anterior and inferior MIs and digoxin toxicity. However, it can occur among healthy elderly people as a result of degenerative changes in the AV node (Leeper 1993, p60). It can also occur among people with high vagal tone, such as athletes.

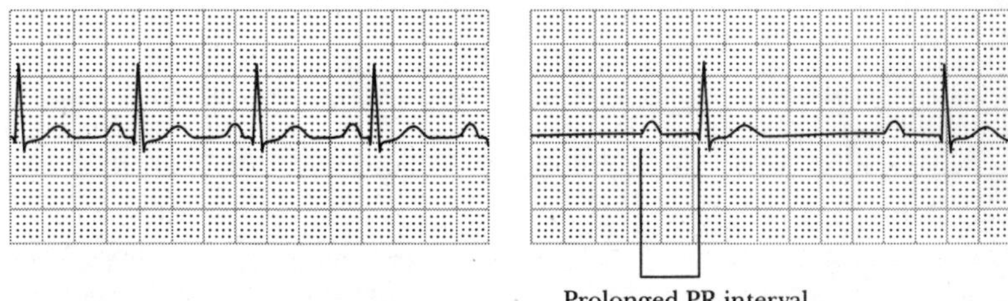

FIGURE 4.26a (left) *Sinus rhythm*
FIGURE 4.26b (right) *First degree AV block*

Characteristics

Rate	38 bpm
Rhythm	regular
P wave	normal (upright, rounded)
PR interval	0.34 seconds
QRS complex	normal
Conduction	there is a delay in the conduction of impulses through the AV node. Ventricular depolarisation is normal

Medical interventions

- Treat underlying cause, such as inferior MI, chronic heart disease or myocarditis
- If rate is slow and patient is symptomatic, treat as in sinus bradycardia
- If necessary, cease drugs causing slow AV node conduction, such as digoxin, beta-blockers or calcium channel blockers and substitute with other drugs

Nursing management

- Monitor and document the arrhythmia
- Monitor vital signs
- Assess for reduced cardiac output
- Administer digoxin with caution as ordered
- Watch for increasing PR interval

SECOND DEGREE AV BLOCK (MOBITZ TYPE I—WENCKEBACH)

Second degree AV block occurs when conduction through the AV node becomes progressively difficult with each successive impulse until, finally, a ventricular beat does not occur. This is characterised by a progressive lengthening of the PR interval. This pattern is repetitive throughout the arrhythmia.

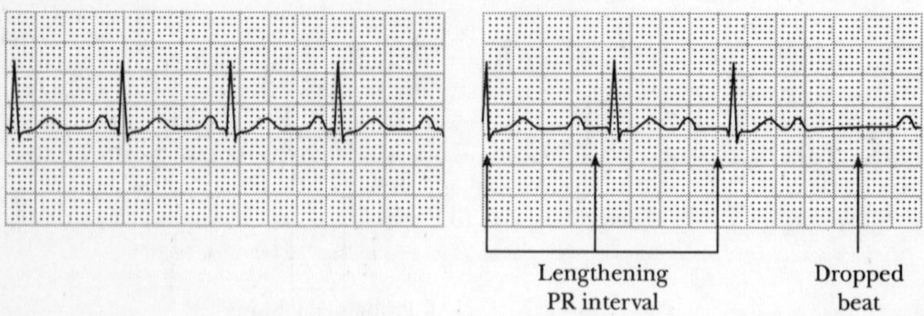

FIGURE 4.27a (left) *Sinus rhythm*

FIGURE 4.27b (right) *Second degree AV block (Mobitz type I)*

Characteristics

Rate	68 bpm (ventricular) in the underlying rhythm; 75 bpm (atrial)
Rhythm	atrial (regular); ventricular (irregular) because of dropped beat
P wave	normal
PR interval	lengthening with each successive beat
QRS complex	normal
Conduction	some of the impulses from the atria are blocked. PR interval gets progressively longer until one P wave is not followed by a QRS complex

Medical interventions

- Treat underlying cause, such as rheumatic fever, inferior MI or digoxin toxicity
- Cease digoxin
- If symptomatic and bradycardic, administer atropine or isoprenaline
- If the underlying rate is tachycardia, determine the cause and treat accordingly (eg pain, fever, anxiety)
- Insert a temporary pacemaker to improve cardiac output

Nursing management

- Monitor and document the arrhythmia
- Watch for more advanced heart block
- Monitor vital signs
- Assess for decreased cardiac output

SECOND DEGREE AV BLOCK (MOBITZ TYPE II)

In this arrythmia two or more atrial impulses are normally conducted to the ventricle, but without warning, the next impulse is blocked. Blocks may occur occas-

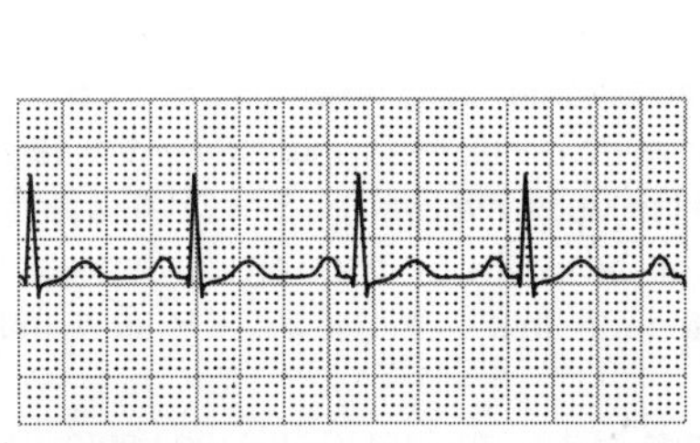

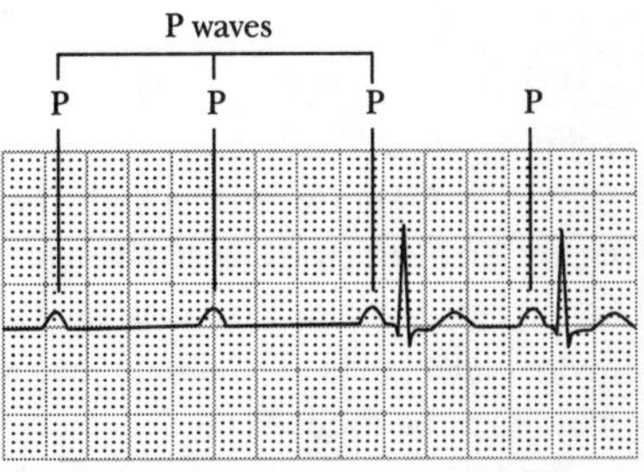

FIGURE 4.28a (left) *Sinus rhythm*
FIGURE 4.28b (right) *Second degree AV block (Mobitz type II)*

sionally or at regular intervals, for example at every third beat (3:1 AV block). Causes of second degree AV block include coronary artery disease, anterior MIs and degenerative changes in the conductive system. This arrhythmia may progress to complete heart block.

Characteristics

Rate	64 bpm (ventricular) is the underlying rhythm
Rhythm	irregular with varying degrees of block
P wave	there are three P waves to one QRS complex. PP intervals are regular
PR interval	0.16 seconds (absent in blocked beats)
QRS complex	0.08 seconds; some dropped complexes
T wave	normal when present (absent in blocked beats)
Conduction	third atrial impulse is conducted through the ventricles

Medical interventions

- Treat underlying cause, such as MI or coronary artery disease.
- Check serum level of digoxin as block may be due to toxicity
- Discontinue digoxin if heart rate is slow or patient is symptomatic
- Administer atropine or isoprenaline
- Temporary pacemaker may be required if patient is symptomatic

Nursing management

- Monitor and document the arrhythmia
- Monitor vital signs
- Assess haemodynamic status, particularly low cardiac output
- Assist in the insertion of pacemaker

THIRD DEGREE AV BLOCK

Third degree AV block (or complete heart block) results when all the impulses above the AV node are blocked. Therefore, no impulse is conducted to the ventricles. To overcome this situation (and if the block involves the SA node), a junctional rhythm arises. However, if the block is below the SA node an idioventricular rhythm takes over. The danger associated with this rhythm is that it is slow and may lead to a reduced cardiac output.

The SA node continues to pace the atria at a normal rate while the ventricles beat at a much slower rate. The P waves and QRS complexes occur at regular intervals, but they are independent of each other.

Blocks occurring above the SA node are associated with inferior MIs and digoxin toxicity. Blocks occurring below the SA node are caused by degenerative changes to the conduction system.

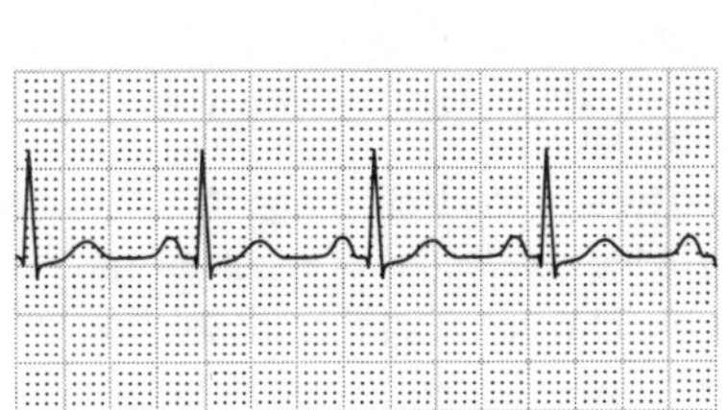

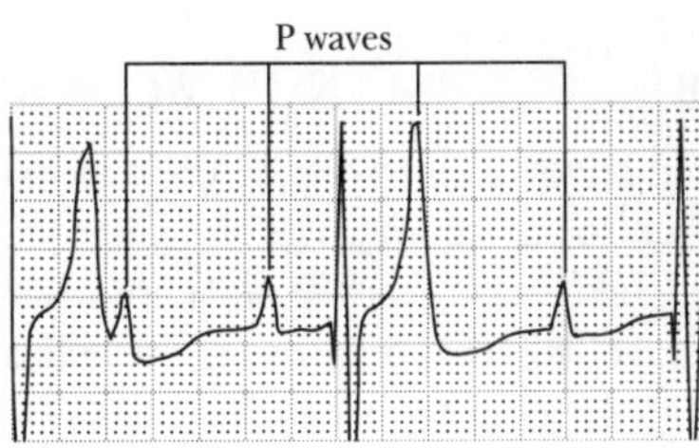

FIGURE 4.29a (left) *Sinus rhythm*
FIGURE 4.29b (right) *Third degree AV block*

Characteristics

Rate	Atrial rate (normally 60–100 bpm) is faster than the ventricular rate. If the ventricular pacemaker originates from the junctional tissue (40–60 bpm); from the Purkinje system (20–40 bpm)
Rhythm	atrial and ventricular rhythms are independent of each other and are regular
P wave	normal (pointed configuration)
PR interval	absent (P waves bear no relationship to the QRS complex)
QRS complex	usually depends on the site of the pacemaker. Wider QRS (greater than 0.20 seconds) if the pacemaker originated from the Purkinje system
Conduction	the atria and the ventricles have an independent pacemaker so that there is no relationship between the two

Medical interventions

- Treat underlying cause, such as acute MIs, ischaemic heart disease, myocarditis or digoxin toxicity
- Assess digoxin serum level and cease when necessary
- Administer atropine or isoprenaline
- Insert temporary pacemaker to improve cardiac output

Nursing management

- Monitor and document the arrhythmia
- Monitor haemodynamic status

- Watch for signs and symptoms of reduced cardiac output
- Monitor tolerance to arrhythmia
- Assist in the insertion of temporary pacemaker

BUNDLE BRANCH BLOCKS

left bundle branch block, right bundle branch block

Bundle branch blocks (BBBs) are the second type of conduction disorders. Bundle branch blocks occur where there is a delay in the conduction of impulses through one of the main branches of the bundle of His (either the right or the left branches). As a consequence, the respective ventricles affected by the BBB are activated abnormally by the impulses coming through the interventricular septum. This abnormal conduction gives rise to a widened QRS complex (greater than 0.12 seconds) as it takes longer for the impulse to travel around the blocked branch. Changes in the ST segment and T wave occur because of the widened QRS complex. A 12 lead ECG is the only way to determine whether the block occurs in the right or left bundle branch. The best leads to view are the chest leads V_1 and V_6.

RIGHT BUNDLE BRANCH BLOCK

In right bundle branch block (RBBB; refer to Figure 4.30) the following takes place: (1) the initial impulse activates the interventricular septum; (2) the left bundle

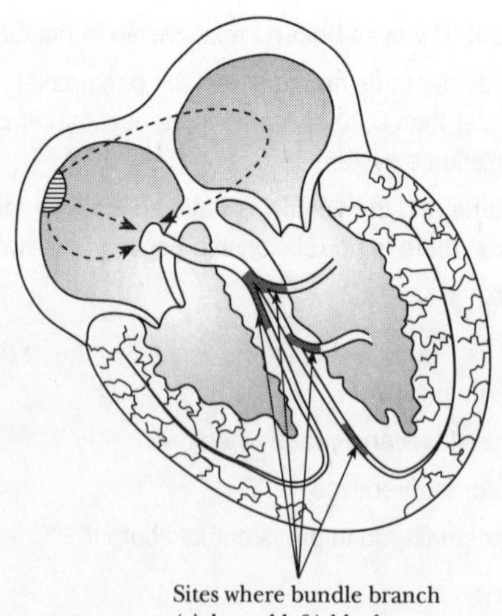

FIGURE 4.30 *Pathway for bundle branch block arrhythmias*

branch stimulates the ventricle to depolarise; and (3) the impulse is transmitted across the septum below the level of the block.

Using the chest lead V1 and V6 on the 12 lead ECG, RBBB is characterised by:

- a small R wave in V_1 and a small Q wave in V_6
- a large S wave in V_1 and a large R wave in V_6
- a second large R wave in V_1 and a deep, wide S wave in V_6.

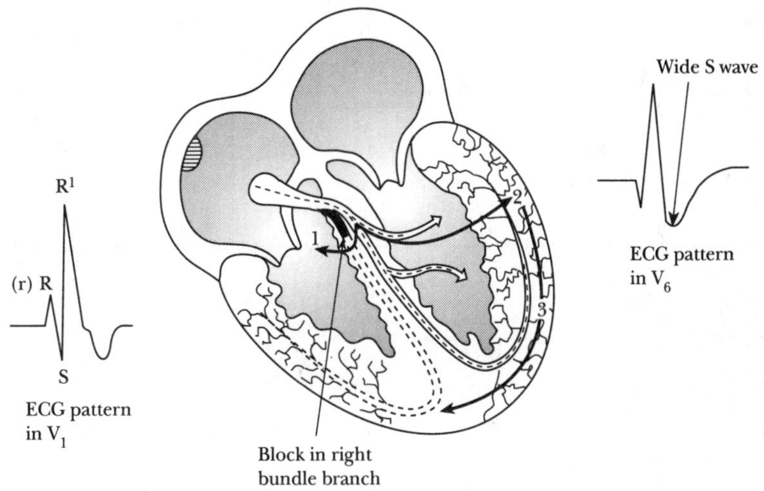

FIGURE 4.31 *Right bundle branch block with characteristic ECG features*

Causes of RBBB include right ventricular hypertrophy, anterior MIs, pulmonary embolism and cardiomyopathy. They can also occur in individuals with 'normal' hearts.

Medical interventions

- Usually no treatment is required, but after an acute MI temporary pacing may be indicated as a preventative measure against the development of arrhythmias

Nursing management

- Document arrhythmia and monitor for further changes

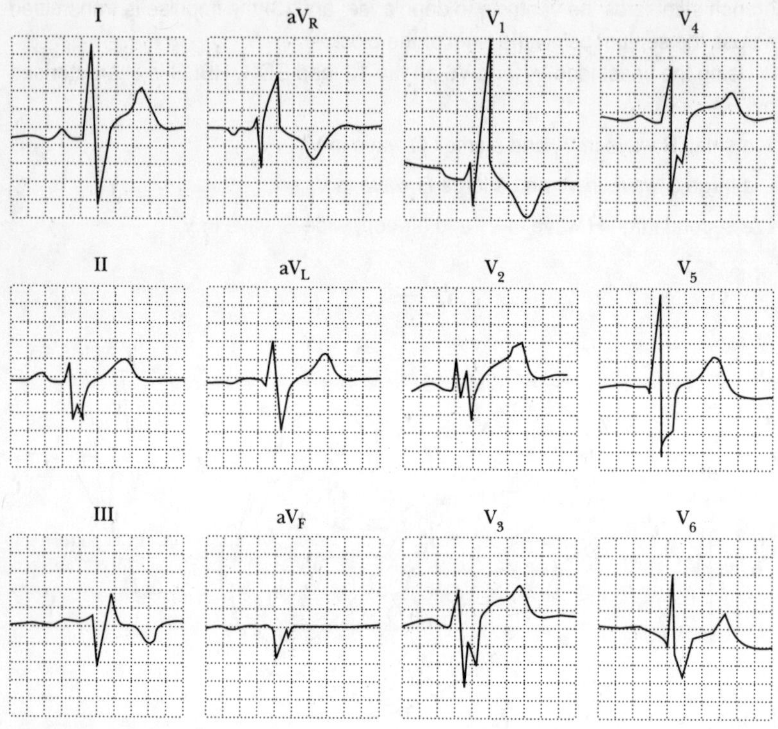

FIGURE 4.32 *A 12 lead ECG of a right bundle branch block. Note that the activation of both ventricles in sequence from the left to the right causes an initial small R wave and a broad complex with a late R wave in* V_1*, giving the triphasic RSR ECG pattern and an S wave in* V_6*. The underlying rhythm is sinus tachycardia with a rate of 130 bpm.*

Source Hampton 1992, p 34

LEFT BUNDLE BRANCH BLOCK

In a left bundle branch block (LBBB) activation of the left ventricle results from conduction of the impulse which spreads from the right ventricle through the interventricular septum of the left bundle branch below the level of the block. The following events occur when the left bundle branch is blocked.

A LBBB may involve part of the main left bundle. It may also involve the anterior and posterior fascicles.

Using the chest leads V_1 and V_6 on the 12 lead ECG, LBBB is characterised by:

- a wide and slurred QS complex in V_1
- a wide and slurred R, rSR or RsR complex in V_6

- no q waves in the septal leads
- the QRS complex being greater than 0.12 seconds because the ventricles do not depolarise simultaneously. This shape poses difficulties when interpreting MIs.
- T wave inversion.

Causes of LBBB include MIs, valvular heart disease and hypertension.

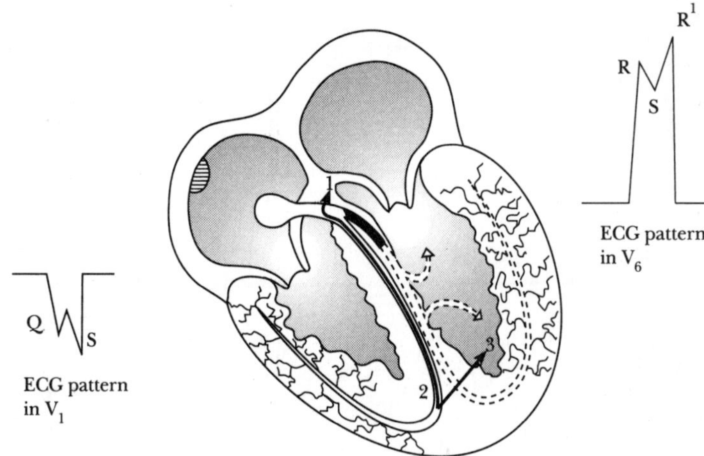

FIGURE 4.33 *Left bundle branch block (characterised in V_6 as an 'M' pattern) with characteristic ECG features*

Non-life-threatening arrhythmias	Life-threatening arrhythmias
Sinus bradycardia*	Sinus arrest
Sinus tachycardia*	Paroxysmal atrial tachycardia
Sinus arrhythmia	Mobitz II heart block
Wandering pacemaker	Third degree AV block
Premature atrial ectopic beats	Idioventricular rhythm
Atrial flutter*	Ventricular ectopic beats
Atrial fibrillation*	Ventricular tachycardia
Junctional rhythm	Ventricular fibrillation
Nonparoxysmal junctional tachycardia*	Ventricular standstill
Paroxysmal junctional tachycardia*	
Accelerated idioventricular rhythm	
First degree heart block	
Bundle branch block*	

* *Under certain conditions these arrhythmias can become life-threatening*

TABLE 4.1 *Summary of arrhythmias*

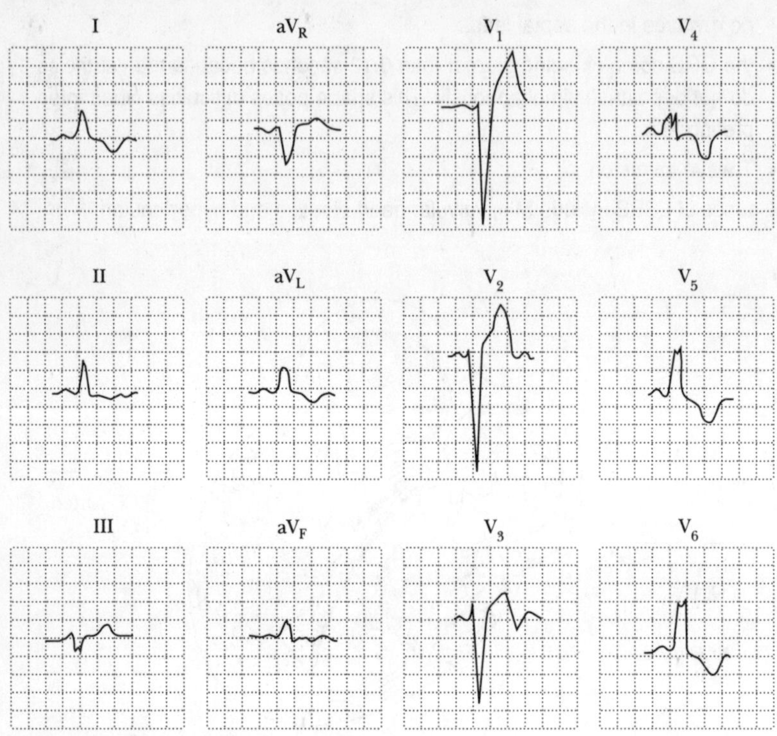

FIGURE 4.34 *A 12 lead ECG of a left bundle branch block. The anterior and posterior fascicles of the left bundle branch fail to conduct impulses through the ventricles, causing a very broad complex that is negative in V_1 and positive in V_6. Note the ECG patterns on these two precordial leads. You will notice a very broad deep S wave on the anterior chest leads and a broad R wave on the lateral chest leads. You will also see the typical 'M' pattern in the LBBB on the ECG.*

Source Hampton 1992, p 35

Arrhythmia	Atrial rate (bpm)	Ventricular rate (bpm)
Sinus bradycardia	40–60	40–60
Sinus tachycardia	100–150	100–150
Sinus arrhythmia	60–100	60–100 (varies with breathing)
Wandering pacemaker	60–100	60–100
Atrial tachycardia*	160–200	50–200
Atrial flutter	250–400	60–160 (depends on number of atrial impulses)
Atrial fibrillation	400–500	120–150 (can have slower rate)
Junctional rhythm	40–60	40–60
Idioventicular rhythm	unable to determine	30–40
Ventricular tachycardia	unable to determine	100–200
Ventricular fibrillation	unable to determine	unable to determine

**Also referred to as supraventricular tachycardia*

TABLE 4.2 *Heart rates of basic arrhythmias*

EXERCISES — CARDIAC RHYTHM INTERPRETATION

Exercise 1

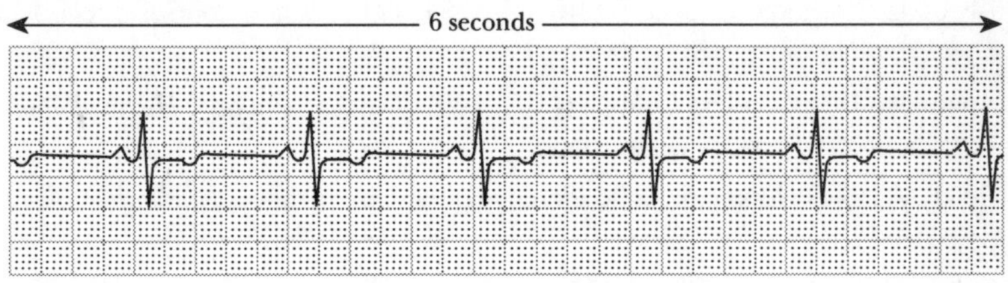

What are the characteristics of the above cardiac rhythm?

1 Rate

2 Rhythm

3 P wave

4 PR interval

5 QRS complex

6 ST segment

7 T wave

8 Interpretation

Exercise 2

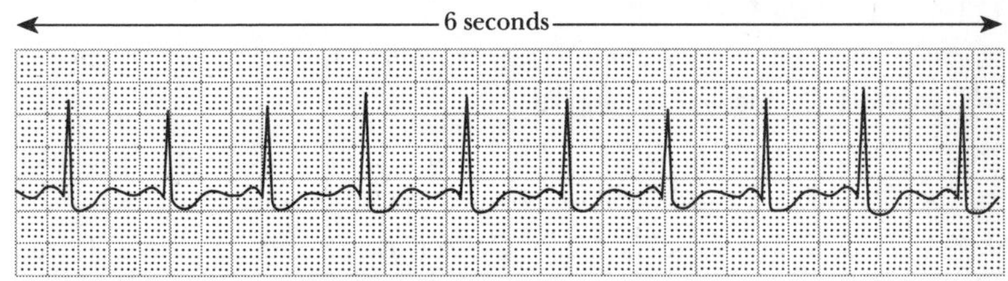

What are the characteristics of the above cardiac rhythm?

1 Rate

2 Rhythm

3 P wave

4 PR interval

5 QRS complex

6 ST segment

7 T wave

8 Interpretation

REFERENCES

Armstrong, M 1985, *Electrocardiograms. A Systematic Method of Reading Them*, 5th edn, John Wrights & Sons Ltd, Bristol

Atwood, S, Stanton, C & Storey, J 1990, *Introduction to Basic Cardiac Dysrhythmias*, Mosby, St Louis

Australian Resuscitation Council (ARC) 1993, *Cardiopulmonary Resuscitation*, Fergies Colour Printers, Queensland

Boltz, M 1994, 'Nurses guide to identifying cardiac rhythms', *Nursing 94*, April, pp 54–5

Bullock, B L & Rosendahl, P P 1992, *Pathophysiology: Adaptation and Alteration in Function*, 3rd edn, J B Lippincott Company, Philadelphia

Camm, A J & Ward, D E 1993, 'Treatment of tachycardia: Cardioversion, defibrillation and pacemakers', *Medicine International*, vol 21, no 11, pp 442–52

Connover, M B 1984, *Exercises in Diagnosing ECG Tracings*, Mosby, St Louis

Connover, M 1990, *Pocket Guide to Electrocardiography*, 2nd edn, Mosby, St Louis

Hamilton, H K 1984, *Nurses Clinical Library: Cardiovascular Disorders*, Springhouse Corporation, Pennsylvania

Hampton, J R 1986, *The ECG Made Easy*, 3rd edn, Churchill Livingstone, London

Hampton, J R 1992, *The ECG Made Easy*, 4th edn, Churchill Livingstone, London

Holloway, N M 1993, *Nursing the Critically Ill Adult*, 4th edn, Addison-Wesley Publishing Company, Redding

Hudak, C M & Lohr, T 1986 *Critical Care Nursing: A Holistic Approach*, 4th edn, J B Lippincott Company, Philadelphia

Hudak, C M, Barbara, M, Gallo, J J & Benz, J 1990, *Critical Care Nursing: A Holistic Approach*, J B Lippincott Company, Philadelphia

Julian, D C & Cowan, J C 1992, *Cardiology*, 6th edn, Bailliere Tindall, Philadelphia

Leeper, B 1993, *Arrhythmia Recognition in Deciphering Difficult ECGs. Advanced Skills*, Springhouse Corporation, Pennsylvania

Meltzer, L E, Pinneo, R & Kitchell, J R 1983, *Intensive Coronary Care: A Manual for Nurses*, 4th edn, Robert J Brady Company, Maryland

Meola, D & Walker, V 1987, 'Responding quickly to tachyarrhythmias', *Nursing*, November, pp 34–41

Noone, J 1992, *Arrhythmia Interpretation: A Workbook for Nurses*, Springhouse Corporation, Pennsylvania

Oh, T E 1990, *Intensive Care Manual*, 3rd edn, Butterworths, Sydney

Owens, M & Daniel, J 1993, 'I.V. magnesium sulphate in the treatment of ventricular tachycardia and acute myocardial infarction', *Critical Care Nurse,* vol 13, no 6, December, pp 83–5

Rowlands, D J 1980, *Understanding Electrocardiography: A New Approach*, Imperial Chemical Industries and Pharmaceutical Division, England

Schamroth, L 1982, *An Introduction to Electrocardiography*, 6th edn, Blackwell Scientific Publications, Melbourne

Shaw, D B 1993, 'Bradycardia, sinus node disease, sinoatrial dysfunction and heart block', *Middle Eastern Education*, Medicine International, vol 21, no 11, pp 446–52

Scherer, J C 1992, *Introductory Clinical Pharmacology*, 4th edn, J B Lippincott Company, Philadelphia

Stillwell, S B 1992, *Mosby's Critical Care Nursing Reference*, Mosby, St Louis

Strawn, R M & Stewart, B P 1993, *Ready Reference for Critical Care*, Jones and Bartlett Publishers, Boston

Van Meter, M & Levine, P G 1982, *Reading ECGs Correctly*, Nursing Skillbook Series, Springhouse Corporation, Pennsylvania

Vinsant, M O & Spence, M I 1989, *Commonsense Approach to Coronary Care: A Program Approach*, 5th edn, Mosby, St Louis

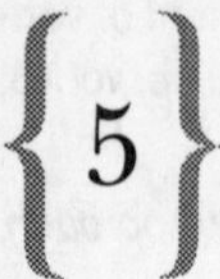

NURSING MANAGEMENT OF PATIENTS WITH ARRHYTHMIAS

OBJECTIVES

After working through this chapter you should be able to:

- identify the factors that place a patient at risk for developing arrhythmias
- discuss the nursing management of patients who develop arrhythmias
- outline the nurse's role and responsibilities during cardioversion and emergency defibrillation
- discuss the indications for using a cardiac pacemaker and describe the nursing care required for patients undergoing treatment with a pacemaker
- discuss alternative interventions which may be used in the management of arrhythmias

KEY WORDS

advanced life support (ALS)
antiarrhythmic drugs
arrhythmia
asynchronised
AV sequential
basic life support (BLS)
bipolar
cardiopulmonary resuscitation (CPR)
cardioversion
defibrillation
demand pacing electrode
joule
microshock
nursing diagnosis
pacemaker
pacing catheter
pulse generator
synchronised
unipolar

Changes are taking place constantly in the health care industry, not just in research and technology, but also in the area of clinical practice. This chapter provides a general guide for assessing arrhythmias and methods of intervention. Discussed also is care for patients who undergo defibrillation, cardioversion and cardiac pacing.

CRITICAL INCIDENT

> *It was 10 am and time to do the next set of observations. I approached Mr Evans in bed 2. He had been admitted during the night with an anterior myocardial infarction. While palpating his radial pulse, I decided to check his cardiac monitor and, as I did, I watched it change from sinus rhythm to ventricular fibrillation. Quickly, I glanced back to my patient's face. His head had already rolled to one side and he was making a gutteral noise in his throat. I snatched the thermometer from his mouth, removed the pillows from behind his back and pushed the emergency button. I laid Mr Evans flat on the bed and reached for the bag and mask, turning the oxygen supply to 12 litres. I checked his breathing and gave him several breaths via the mask. Within a matter of seconds, the ICU team was there and my patient was defibrillated successfully. Within a few minutes Mr Evans was breathing spontaneously. He opened his eyes and immediately became alarmed. I told him what had happened. He nodded his head, became relaxed and said, 'Well, I'm glad I'm still here'.* (E Nash's experience)

Incidents such as this occur every day in specialist units and ward areas. Therefore, it is important for you to be able to recognise the warning signs of an impending arrhythmia and be able to prevent them from becoming a life-threatening situation for the patient. You should also be proficient at basic and advanced life support skills in order to function well in emergency situations.

ASSESSMENT

Initial assessment of the patient in the form of observation should be commenced from the moment the patient arrives in the ward area. As the patient is transferred from the trolley to the bed, the nurse can assess the patient's behavioural and physical responses to the arrhythmia. Generally, most patients feel a loss of control and being in a strange environment makes them feel isolated. While caring for a patient experiencing any arrhythmia, it is important to stay with them, provide them with reassurance and to assess the situation constantly. As soon as the patient has settled and is feeling more comfortable, you can then perform a complete assessment of the patient.

HISTORY

A systematic, continuous and complete data collection about the past and present health status of the patient can assist you in planning the nursing care and subsequent evaluation of the care given. The patient's condition will determine what history can be recorded and, until their situation stabilises, it is advisable to take the most essential history of the patient, especially their current health problems. Once the patient's condition becomes stable, a sociocultural and complete family history can be taken. Each cardiac unit will have its own cardiac assessment tool that you can use which you must be familiar with, however, you must remember to ask the patient for the following history.

Previous illnesses

- History of cardiac disease
- History of respiratory disease
- Whether there have been previous hospitalisations
- Previous surgery
- Whether the patient is currently prescribed medication, such as cardiac medication, antihypertensive drugs, diuretics or bronchodilators used for the treatment of asthma — these may have potent arrhythrogenic properties

Rationale

Arrhythmias are usually a consequence of underlying physical problems, cardiac disorders or may be associated with drug intake. Although it is not your responsibility to pinpoint exactly the cause of the arrhythmia, background information given by the patient will alert the nurse to the possibility of its cause.

Family history

- Cardiac diseases, hypertension, diabetes mellitus, renal disorders, cancer, obesity, cerebrovascular disorders, asthma, vascular disorders (varicositis and atherosclerosis and elevated cholesterol levels). Information should be elicited about the father, mother, brothers, sisters and both maternal and paternal grandparents

Rationale

Some diseases are hereditary. Heart disease is a well-known familial disease either from the first or second generation (eg sudden cardiac death syndrome).

Social history

- Coffee and tea intake, alcohol intake and smoking
- Type and level of exercise or any other type of relaxation and leisure activities, including rest and sleep patterns

- Occupation
- Eating habits
- Cultural beliefs about health and illness, including religious beliefs

Rationale

Sympathetic nervous system stimulants such as caffeine, alcohol and nicotine, can cause arrhythmias. Eliciting information about the patient's habits will help you plan your health education strategy. Cultural beliefs about health and illness will also enable you to plan appropriate culturally congruent care to facilitate the patient's compliance to treatment and medication.

Subjective complaints

- Chest pain (type — stabbing, squeezing, pressure, burning, heavy, dull, choking, intermittent; location — mid-sternum, radiating to left arm, jaw; onset; duration; what relieves it; accompanying symptoms)
- Shortness of breath
- Palpitations
- Diaphoresis
- Physical and emotional experiences, such as lethargy, confusion, blackouts, dizziness, anxiety and restlessness

Note: each of these complaints, especially pain, must be further assessed according to precipitating factors; quality of each symptom and the quantity or frequency of its occurrence; factors which helped relieve the symptoms; accompanying symptoms; and length or duration of each symptom experienced (Ignativiticus & Bayne 1991, p 2131).

Rationale

Subjective complaints consist of symptoms which the patient alone experiences. Acute pain is frightening and chronic pain is exhausting. Pain is difficult to define but, according to McCaffrey and Beebe (1987, p 7), 'Pain is whatever the experiencing person says it is, existing whenever the experiencing person says it does'. It is therefore important to elicit the details of the symptom experienced for you to understand fully what the patient is experiencing in order to plan appropriate nursing interventions. For example, pain stimulates the sympathetic nervous system, resulting in increased heart rate, respiratory rate and peripheral vasoconstriction.

PHYSICAL ASSESSMENT

Physical assessment is performed to check the patient's history. It can also be used as a base to evaluate the patient's progress in the days following admission. While conducting the physical assessment you should bear in mind that arrhythmias can lead to a decrease in cardiac output because of impaired ventricular function. You should also take note that if the assessment is performed systematically, signs and symptoms relating to this condition should be detected immediately. Record measurements (such as blood pressure and heart rate) which reflect not only cardiac function, but also cerebral, coronary and renal functions (Ignativiticus & Bayne 1991, p 2131).

The following focus assessment on a patient with an arrhythmia will be covered in this chapter.

RESPIRATORY ASSESSMENT

- Inspect the rate, depth, rhythm and effort of respiration — the character of respiratory movements may reveal specific ventilatory disorders or disease states. Alterations in respiration may also accompany other symptoms the patient is experiencing, such as chest pain (Bates 1991, p 242; Potter 1990, p 49).
- Inspect for any chest deformities and asymmetry of the chest wall (eg kyphoscoliosis can alter normal lung compliance).

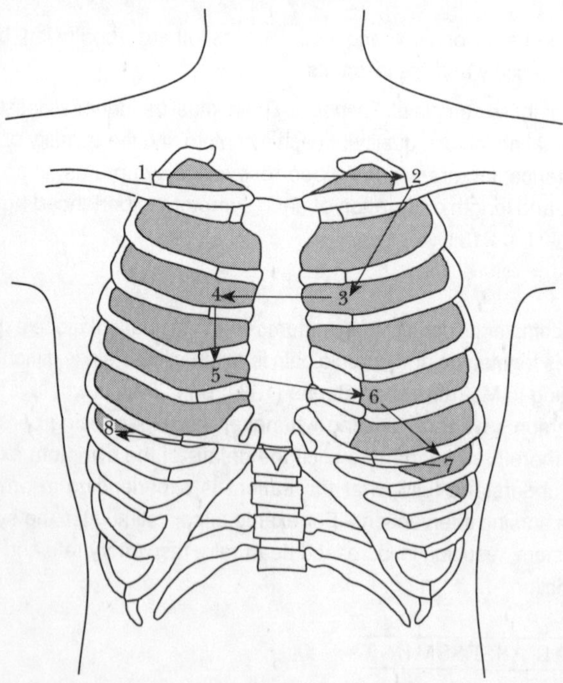

FIGURE 5.1 *Sequence for thoracic percussion and auscultation of the anterior chest wall*

- Palpate the chest to determine any tenderness. Assess chest expansion and detect presence of fremitus (palpable vibrations transmitted through the lung tissue to the chest wall when the patient speaks).
- Percuss both sides of the anterior and posterior chest comparing both sides all the time. Dullness will be heard over solid organ areas, such as the liver or over fluid-filled areas (eg pleural effusion). Resonance is heard over the air-filled lungs (Bates 1991, p 247).
- Listen (with the use of the diaphragm of the stethoscope) for breath sounds or air flow on both sides of the anterior and posterior chest. *Bronchial sounds* are high-pitched sounds heard over the trachea mostly during expirations. *Bronchovesicular sounds* are moderately pitched sounds heard over the main bronchus during inspiration and expiration. *Vesicular sounds* are soft, low-pitched sounds heard over the lung tissue mostly during inspiration. Listen carefully for the presence of *adventitious* sounds such as: *rales* (crackling sounds heard during inspiration as a result of alveolar reinflation); *rhonchi* (coarse sounds heard during expiration as a result of the presence of fluid in the larger airways); *wheezes* (musical sounds heard during inspiration

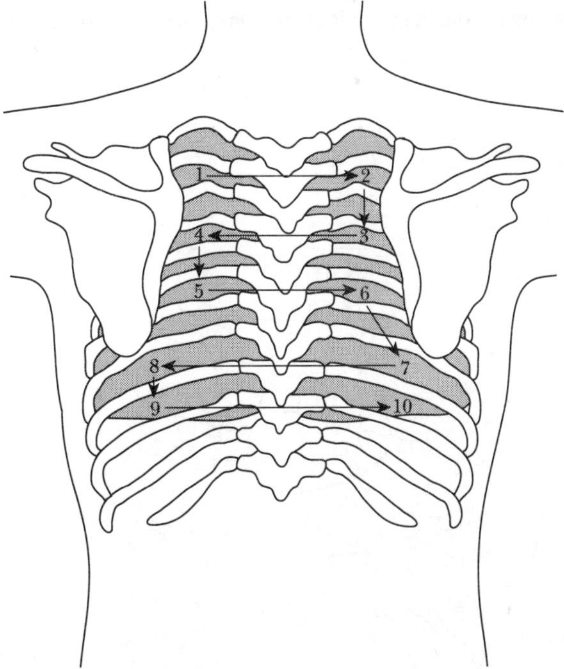

FIGURE 5.2 *Sequence for thoracic percussion and auscultation of the posterior chest wall*

and expiration as a result of bronchospasm); or decreased breath sounds on the right and left upper lobes, right middle lobes and right and left lower lobes. Crackles and wheezes indicate lung congestion (Bates 1991, pp 249–59; Fuller & Schaller-Ayres 1994, p 249; Potter 1990, pp 508–10; Smeltzer & Bare 1992, pp 119–21; Taylor, Lillis & LeMone 1989, pp 455–9).

Areas for percussion and auscultation of the anterior and posterior chest wall are shown in Figures 5.1 and 5.2 on pages 102 and 103 respectively. Follow the sequential order during your assessment.

CARDIAC ASSESSMENT

- Palpate the radial pulse and note the rhythm. If the cardiac rhythm is irregular, the apex beat should be auscultated and counted for one full minute.
- Inspect the anterior chest region and note the size and shape of the thoracic wall. You will be able to determine the location of the heart by the presence of the apical pulse.
- Palpate for pulsations. The apical impulse can be palpated at the left fifth intercostal space at the mid-clavicular line. Observe for any abnormal pulsations over the aortic (second intercostal space, right of sternum), pulmonic (second intercostal space, left of sternum), tricuspid (between the fourth and

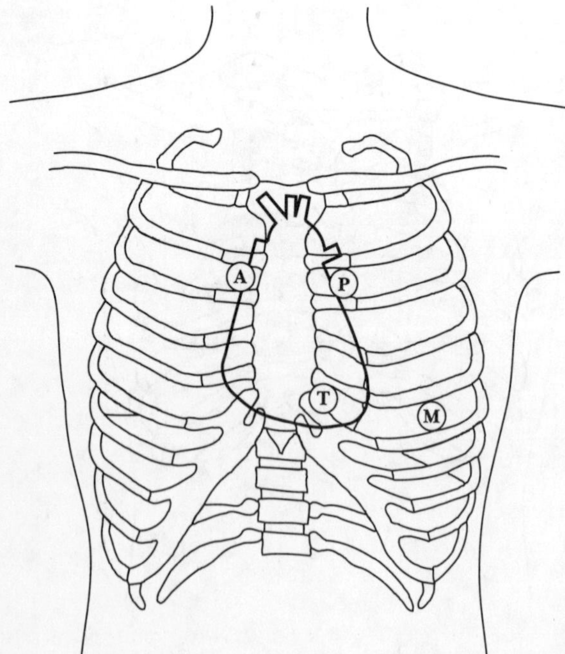

A = aortic area
P = pulmonic area
T = tricuspid area
M = mitral area

FIGURE 5.3 *Landmarks for assessing heart sounds*

fifth intercostal space, left of sternum) and mitral areas (fifth intercostal space, left of sternum, mid-clavicular line; Bates 1991; Smeltzer & Bare 1992).

- Percuss the heart's border to determine the size of the heart (dull sounds will be heard over the heart as in the liver).
- Listen to the heart sounds to detect normal heart sounds and extra heart sounds. Use the diaphragm of the stethoscope to listen for heart sounds. Begin with the aortic area, then the pulmonic area, then the tricuspid area and lastly the mitral area. Refer to Figure 5.3 on page 104 to guide you in assessing the position of these areas.

The heart sounds occur in relation to the cardiac cycle. S1 is the closing of the mitral and tricuspid valve and will be heard as a 'lub' sound; S2 is the closing of the aortic and pulmonary valve after the ventricles empty and will be heard as a 'dub' sound. Each combination of S1 and S2 counts for one heart beat. In auscultating for S3 and S4, use the bell of your stethoscope and place it over the mitral area and position the patient on their left side. S3 (or ventricular gallop rhythm) is normal in children and adults under 30 years of age. If S3 is present in people over 30 years, it may signify volume overload in the ventricle. You will most likely hear this murmur in patients with congestive cardiac failure, valvular heart disease and cardiomyopathy. S4 (or atrial gallop rhythm) results from increased resistance to ventricular filling during atrial contractions (Bates 1987). For S3 and S4 it is suggested that you use the bell of the stethoscope as these sounds are low-pitched. The presence of S3 and S4 indicates reduced compliance of the myocardium, resulting in decreased cardiac output (Bates 1991, p 313; Fuller & Schaller-Ayers 1994, pp 243–7; Potter 1990, pp 126–7; Smeltzer & Bare 1992; Taylor, Lillis & LeMone 1989, pp 459–62).

Murmurs are 'created by the terminal flow of blood' (Smeltzer & Bare 1992, p 627) and can be high-, medium- or low-blowing, rumbling or musical sounds. The location for listening to these sounds are the same as for listening to the heart sounds shown in Figure 5.3. Note the *timing*, *location*, *pitch* and *quality* of the murmurs. Murmurs can be a result of damage to the heart valves, such as incompetence or stenosis (Bates 1991, pp 316–17; Potter 1990, pp 127–8; Taylor, Lillis & LeMone 1989), or from ventricular and atrial septal defects.

VASCULAR ASSESSMENT

Each time the left ventricle ejects blood into the aorta, pressure waves are transmitted to the arterial system. Under normal conditions strong palpable pulses will be felt at the carotid, femoral, brachial, radial, popliteal, posterior tibial and dorsalis pedis arteries.

- Inspect the hands, arms and legs. Note the colour of the skin and nail beds, temperature, skin turgor and texture, presence of any skin lesions, oedema or clubbing of the fingers, and venous patterns. Normally, venous patterns should be flat and barely visible. Clubbing is associated with cor pulmonale and bacterial endocarditis.

- Check the capillary refill by depressing and releasing the nail beds and note the time it takes for colour to return. This should occur in less than one second and gives an indication of peripheral perfusion and cardiac output (Underhill et al 1989, p 260).

- Palpate the radial and apical pulses. These are taken for one full minute. Check for any irregularity in the rhythm as well as the presence of pulse deficits — the strength of the pulse felt at the radial artery indicates the volume of blood ejected with each contraction of the heart (Fuller & Schaller-Ayers 1989, pp 459–63; Potter 1990, pp 131–2).

- Record the blood pressure from both arms — this provides information about the patient's haemodynamic status, such as cardiac output and systemic vascular resistance.

- Palpate the arteries (carotid, radial, ulnar, brachial, popliteal, posterior tibial and dorsalis pedis) gently with your index and middle finger. With the exception of the carotid arteries, all other peripheral arteries can be palpated at the same time to compare the left from the right side. Note the rate, rhythm and elasticity of the vessel wall and the strength of pulses. Carotid arteries must be palpated one at a time and as lightly as possible to avoid carotid sinus stimulation.

- Measure the jugular venous pressure. The internal jugular vein can be seen on both sides of the neck just above the clavicle. Normally veins are flat, but if it is elevated and very distinct, it may be associated with right-side heart failure. The jugular venous pressure (JVP) can be measured by the following steps (Bates 1991, pp 286–8; Fuller & Schaller-Ayres 1994, pp 255–6; Taylor, Lillis & LeMone 1989, p 976).

  a Place the patient on their back with the head of the bed elevated 30°.

  b Turn the patient's head to the left.

  c With the aid of an angle poise light positioned so that the neck is partially shaded, look for the 'flickering' pulse of the internal jugular vein.

  d Place a metric ruler vertically on top of the sternal angle (manubrial joint). Place another metric ruler horizontal to the first ruler, with its lower edge placed against the highest point (meniscus) of the pulse.

  e Read from the vertical ruler the approximate height of the JVP, bearing in mind that the sternal angle is already 4 cm above the right atrium. The normal JVP should be less than 3–4 cm.

Refer to Figure 5.4 to illustrate this procedure.

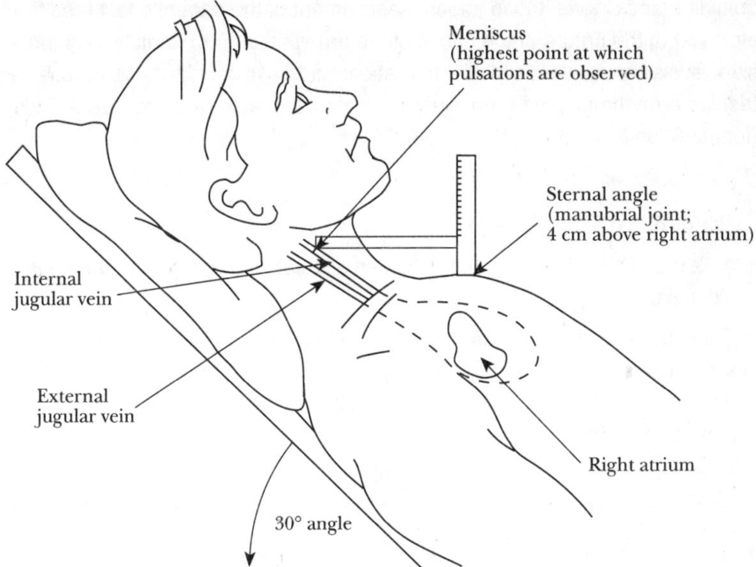

FIGURE 5.4 *Jugular venous pressure measurement*

NEUROLOGICAL ASSESSMENT

Since alteration in tissue perfusion, brought about by a decrease in cardiac output during arrhythmia, affects cerebral function, simple assessment of the patient's neurological status has to be undertaken. Sometimes an arrhythmia may cause a temporary loss of consciousness due to lack of cerebral blood flow. After the arrhythmic episode you should complete the following tasks:

- assess the patient's level of consciousness, note the level of arousal and state of orientation to person, time and place
- check voluntary movement of each extremity by giving simple and specific commands
- assess the strength of the upper extremities by asking the patient to squeeze your fingers.
- assess their strength of the lower extremities by asking the patient to push the feet against your hands
- check pupillary response to light and note size, shape and symmetry of both pupils.

Laboratory findings

It is important for the nurse responsibile to have adequate knowledge about test results, such as serum levels of potassium, calcium, magnesium, digoxin, quinidine and arterial blood gases. Assessment of the patient's test results will alert you to the nature of the cause of the arrhythmia. For example, high potassium levels can cause ventricular fibrillation; acid-base imbalance can cause ventricular arrhythmia; and high digoxin levels can cause first degree AV block (Ignatavicius & Bayne 1991, p 2094).

Other diagnostic tests

1 A 12 lead ECG is recorded to obtain an accurate assessment of the heart's electrical activity.
2 Continuous cardiac monitoring is used to assess the frequency and type of arrhythmias. When interpreting arrhythmias, remember the five points: rate, rhythm, P wave, PR interval and QRS duration (as discussed in Chapters 2 and 4).
3 Other tests, such as telemetry, ambulatory monitoring, electrophysiologic studies and exercise testing, may also be necessary (refer to Chapter 3).

You must be familiar with all these diagnostic tests in order to confidently and competently assist in the preparation and post-procedure care of patients.

Antiarrhythmic drugs

Knowledge of the most commonly used drugs and their indications, dosages, effects and side effects will assist you in evaluating the effectiveness of the drug therapy as well as planning health education for patients and their families.

Antiarrhythmic drugs are classified into four categories according to their effects on cardiac muscle.

Class 1 — reduces the influx of sodium ions during phase 0 of the action potential. They tend to stabilise the cell membrane.

Class 1a — depresses the membrane responsiveness and slows the upstroke of phase 0. ECG features include a prolonged QT interval and a slightly wider QRS complex. Examples include quinidine, procaineamide and disopyramide.

Class 1b — inhibits the fast sodium channels and shortens the action potential. ECG features include a prolonged PR interval and a slightly wider QRS complex. Examples include lignocaine, mexilitene and phenytoin.

Class 1c — inhibits the fast sodium channels and slows the upstroke to phase 0. Drugs in this class also inhibit the conduction to the bundle of His and the Purkinje fibres. ECG features include a prolonged PR interval and QT interval, and a wider QRS complex. Examples include flecainide and encainide.

Class 2 — decreases impulse formation (automaticity in the sinus node), atrial tissue, junctional cells and the Purkinje fibres. ECG features include a slightly prolonged PR interval and a shorter QT interval. Examples include propranolol, arenolol and sotalol.

Class 3 — prolongs the refractory period and the action potential. Drugs in this class also increase the threshold of ventricular fibrillation, making fibrillation more effective. ECG features include a prolonged PR interval, a wider, or normal, QRS complex and a prolonged QT interval. Examples include bretylium tosylate and amiodarone.

Class 4 — blocks the influx of calcium ions across the slow channels in smooth muscle cells. ECG features include an increase in the time duration of the PR interval and a decrease in heart rate. Examples include verapamil and nifedipine (Underhill et al 1989, pp 629–42).

COMMON NURSING DIAGNOSIS

Based on a physical examination and the patient's history, you will have determined the nature and condition of the arrhythmia.

In addition, you may also make the following diagnoses. With each diagnosis, you will be required to perform the necessary nursing interventions in the successful management of the arrhythmia.

1 Anxiety related to knowledge deficit of patient's diagnosis and possible outcomes.
2 Decreased cardiac output related to arrhythmias secondary to impaired pacemaker function or presence of multiple irritable foci.
3 Alteration in tissue perfusion: cardiopulmonary, cerebral, renal, peripheral and gastrointestinal tissue perfusion related to ineffective cardiac pumping and decreased cardiac output.
4 Activity intolerance related to imbalance between oxygen supply and demand secondary to decreased cardiac output.
5 Alteration in comfort related to arrhythmia which may be accompanied by chest pain or discomfort.

Nursing diagnosis 1 Anxiety related to knowledge deficit of patient's diagnosis and possible outcomes.

Goal The patient will understand and accept their disease and will show compliance with the treatment.

Nursing interventions	Rationale
Initiate patient/family education consisting of topics such as • disease process • diet and exercise • how to monitor your own pulse • when to alert the doctor • reasons for taking medications, right time and dosages, common side-effects of antiarrhythmic drugs, such as nausea, vomiting, dizziness and chest discomfort	Prepare patient and family for discharge. Such health education must always be timed and planned appropriately and must always include the family or significant others. Providing the necessary information and knowing the appropriate actions to take during emergencies will help relieve anxiety experienced by the patient and the family.

cont next page

Nursing interventions	Rationale
• implanted pacemaker or cardioverter/defibrillator devices	Refer to the discussion of electrical devices on pages 115–29.
• encourage enrolment in basic life support (BLS) classes to learn basic CPR (for significant others)	
• refer patient to the cardiac rehabilitation program.	Allows the opportunity to talk with other patients with the same problems and concerns under guidance of cardiac rehabilitation team.
Provide the opportunity to verbalise fears. Reassure patient and family. Encourage client to engage in relaxation techniques. Offer spiritual support.	Talking to the patient and family decreases feelings of anxiety. Many patients are frightened because of a variety of reasons which may include a refusal to accept what has happened and uncertainty of their future.

Nursing diagnosis 2 Decreased cardiac output related to arrhythmias secondary to impaired pacemaker function or presence of multiple irritable foci.

Goal The patient will have a cardiac rhythm adequate to maintain a normal cardiac output and maintain haemodynamic stability.

Nursing interventions	Rationale
Record and document vital signs. Some units have the following regime: • half-hourly for the first two hours, then • hourly for 12 hours, then • four-hourly thereafter.	Hypotension and alteration in heart rate may occur especially during the acute episodes of arrhythmia. Widening pulse pressure indicates declining cardiac output.
Assess cardiac monitor patterns (rate and rhythm) by doing the following: • continuous cardiac monitoring • attach hourly rhythm strips on the patient's notes.	Assesses cardiac rate and rhythm regularly. This prevents other complications of arrhythmias, such as those which can lead to cardiac arrest and include VT, VF, and R on T phenomena. It will also determine the effect of drug therapy.
Administer oxygen.	Increases myocardial oxygenation.
Stay with the patient and watch the cardiac monitor. The doctor may need to perform carotid sinus massage to terminate the arrhythmia.	Staying with the patient will help reassure the patient and help decrease the sympathetic response seen in anxiety. Blood pressure and heart rate decreases from vagal stimulation as stretch receptors within the carotid sinus are stimulated (Ignavitacius & Bayne 1991, p 2094).
Administer drugs appropriate to the type of arrhythmia (per doctor's orders). Classification of antiarrhythmic drugs is discussed on pages 108–9.	Drugs are necessary only if the patient is symptomatic. One or more antiarrhythmic drugs may be ordered for the patient. Check correct dosages of drugs and the effects they may have on the cardiac muscles.

cont next page

Nursing interventions	Rationale
For VT administer lignocaine 50–100 mg bolus (or 1 mg/kg), followed by lignocaine infusion at 2–4 g/min initially titrated to the patient's response.	
For VF administer precordial thump only during a witness arrest*. Call for help. Start CPR immediately, starting with BLS. Advanced life support (ALS) is commenced as soon as the arrest team arrives at the scene. Defibrillate at 200–400 joules (if allowed by the hospital or unit director). Follow the hospital protocol for arrest procedures. (Refer to the CPR algorithm in Figures 5.5 and 5.6 for BLS and ALS).	VF results in cardiopulmonary arrest. Emergency treatment of witnessed cardiac arrest requires immediate action. Speed and team work is crucial to the success of resuscitation. The mechanical energy from the precordial thump creates electrical stimulus that can depolarise the heart for witnessed, pulseless arrest. Defibrillation results in complete depolarisation of the myocardium leading to the termination of certain tachyarrhythmias.

*The Australian Resuscitation Council does not recommend the precordial thump highly, nor does it regard it as obsolete (Harrison 1994).

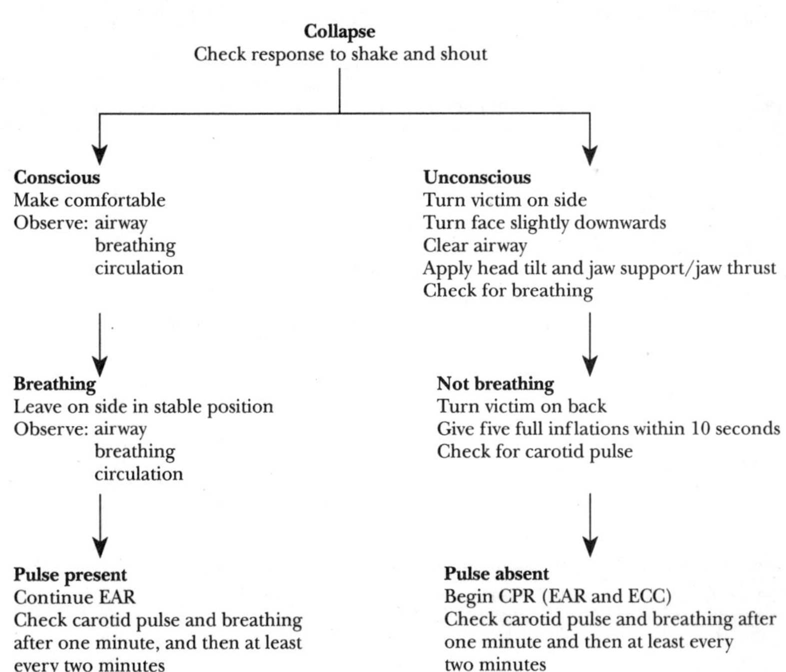

Collapse
Check response to shake and shout
Conscious
Make comfortable
Observe: airway
breathing
circulation
Unconscious
Turn victim on side
Turn face slightly downwards
Clear airway
Apply head tilt and jaw support/jaw thrust
Check for breathing
Breathing
Leave on side in stable position
Observe: airway
breathing
circulation
Not breathing
Turn victim on back
Give five full inflations within 10 seconds
Check for carotid pulse
Pulse present
Continue EAR
Check carotid pulse and breathing
after one minute, and then at least
every two minutes
Pulse absent
Begin CPR (EAR and ECC)
Check carotid pulse and breathing after
one minute and then at least every
two minutes
EAR = Expired Air Resuscitation
ECC = External Cardiac Compression
CPR = Cardiopulmonary Resuscitation

FIGURE 5.5 *Basic life support algorithm*

Source Australian Resuscitation Council 1993, p 2

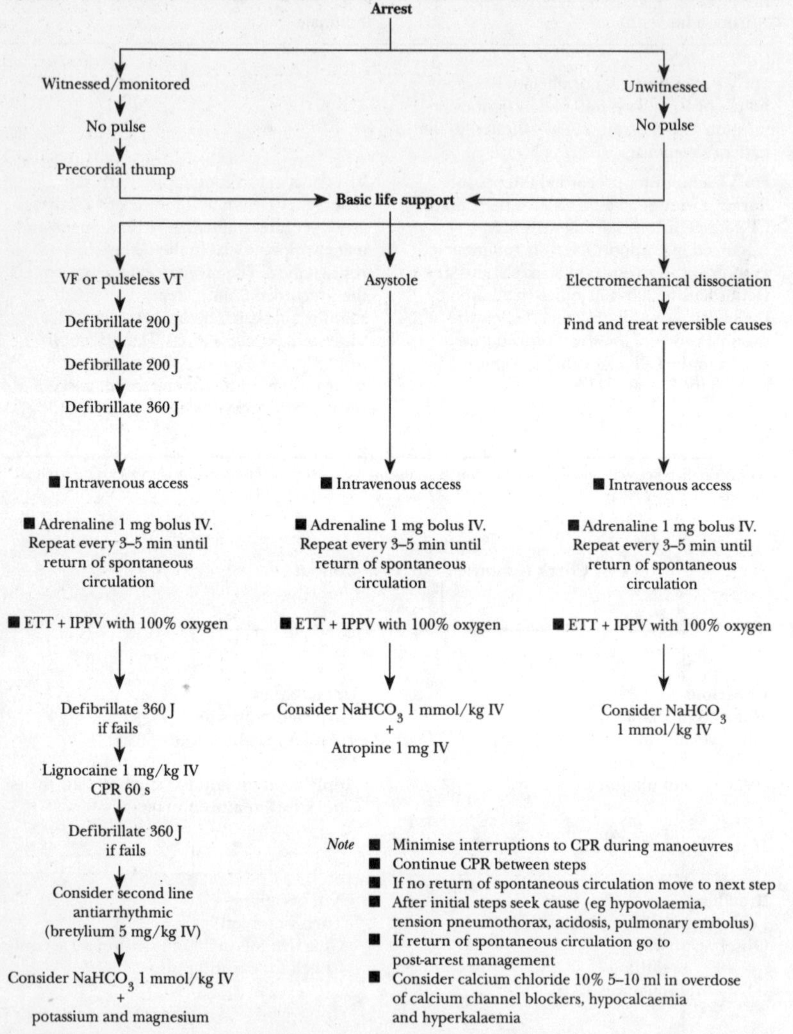

FIGURE 5.6 *Advanced life support algorithm*

Source Adult Advanced Life Support Committee of the Australian Resuscitation Council 1993, pp 616–21.

The algorithms illustrated in Figures 5.5 and 5.6 have been developed to provide uniformity of the practice of BLS and ALS based on the 1992 guidelines of the American Heart Association (AHA) and the European Resuscitation Council (ARC 1993, p 616). The algorithms suggest series of actions to be undertaken by the resuscitator. The patient's ECG rhythm and pulse must be monitored continuously throughout the resuscitation process.

All patients who have a witnessed or unwitnessed cardiac arrest should receive BLS immediately. The precordial thump may be of value while waiting for the arrest team who can defibrillate the patient. However, it is recommended by the ARC that this procedure be initiated only in a witnessed arrest during which the patient is already monitored at the time of the arrhythmia (ARC 1993, p 617).

Nursing diagnosis 3 Alteration in tissue perfusion: cardiopulmonary, cerebral, renal, peripheral and gastrointestinal tissues related to ineffective cardiac pumping and decreased cardiac output.

Goal The patient will maintain adequate tissue perfusion to all vital areas of the body.

Nursing interventions	Rationale
Monitor vital signs (temperature, pulse, respiration and blood pressure) regularly or according to unit's protocol. Continuous cardiac monitoring. Assess level of consciousness, especially during the arrhythmic episodes. Maintain 24-hour fluid balance chart. Monitor patient's intake and output. It may be necessary to restrict fluid intake.	Left ventricular function is usually affected during arrhythmias. Assessment of the cerebral, coronary and renal perfusion can be traced through the presence of hypotension, confusion, chest pain, shortness of breath, jugular vein distension, fatigue and oliguria (Ignatavicius & Bayne 1991, p 2091; Smeltzer & Bare 1992, pp 622–4).
Provide low sodium diet.	Fluid retention is usually associated with the heart's inability to pump blood effectively into systemic circulation. Salt can facilitate water reabsorption.

Nursing diagnosis 4 Activity intolerance related to imbalance between oxygen supply and demand secondary to decreased cardiac output.

Goal The patient will be able to tolerate simple activities that require less energy. The patient will also maintain adequate cardiac output to maintain ventilation and perfusion requirements.

Nursing interventions	Rationale
Space nursing and medical interventions and allow patient to rest in between, especially in the early recovery stage.	Resting decreases demand for oxygen.

cont next page

Nursing interventions	Rationale
Assess respiratory rate, rhythm depth and effort, especially after an activity such as walking around the bed or after having a shower.	The characteristics of the patient's respiration will alert you to the cardiopulmonary status of the patient. Shortness of breath can be due to decreased cardiac output as the demand might be greater than the supply. It can also be associated with pulmonary congestion which may be a complication of heart failure.
Assist the patient as much as possible in all activities. Bed rest may be ordered during the initial stages of hospitalisation. Assess the patient's tolerance to non-strenuous activities.	Complete bed rest decreases demand for myocardial oxygen and relaxes the heart.
Tailor the patient's activities according to their condition. A gradual increase in activity is recommended.	The patient's activities can be increased gradually, depending on your assessment of the cardiopulmonary effects of such activities.

Nursing diagnosis 5 Alteration in comfort related to arrhythmia which may be accompanied by chest pain or discomfort.

Goal The patient will be free from discomfort.

Nursing interventions	Rationale
Administer appropriate analgesics as ordered.	Relieves pain and discomfort as well as severe anxiety related to feeling of impending death, especially if acute pain is experienced.
Provide bed rest until the patient's condition is stable.	Increased oxygen demand which is greater than the supply will potentiate ischaemic episodes to the myocardial tissues.
Restrict flow of visitors to the nearest relatives.	Entertaining lots of visitors can lead to emotional and physical tiredness. Excitement can stimulate the sympathetic nervous system by increasing the heart rate, respiratory rate and blood pressure, resulting in more workload for the heart.
Relieve anxiety or apprehension if present by letting the patient talk about their fears.	Allows the patient time to accept their condition and provides the nurse with the opportunity to keep the patient informed of their progress. Builds better rapport between the patient and nurse.
Offer relaxation techniques, such as music, reading materials or videos.	Provides the patient with a sense of control.

ELECTRICAL THERAPY FOR ARRHYTHMIAS

As a result of continuing research and development, electrical therapy for specific arrhythmias is relatively safe and effective. Three forms of electrical therapy are discussed: *defibrillation*, *cardioversion* and *cardiac pacing*.

DEFIBRILLATION

A defibrillator is a 'device capable of delivering electrical energy to the heart' (Whitford 1990, p 75; see Figure 5.7). Defibrillation is the delivery of a non-synchronised direct current electrical countershock of 200–360 joules which results in complete depolarisation of the myocardium. This leads to the termination of specific tachyarrhythmias, such as ventricular fibrillation. 'Non-synchronised' implies that there is no QRS sensing mechanism operating in the defibrillator as these arrhythmias do not have this ECG complex.

When ventricular fibrillation is confirmed, defibrillation must be carried out immediately by either a doctor or an authorised cardiac nurse specialist. The following procedure is performed.

1 The patient must be in a supine position and connected to the cardiac monitor.

2 Paddles are coated with a conduction paste to prevent electrical burns to the patient's chest. However, some manufacturers provide (pre-packed) defibrillator jel pads.

3 Turn on the defibrillator machine and move the dial to the required energy level. For an adult of average size and weight, 200 joules is recommended (refer to Figure 5.6 on p 112). Depress the charge button on the appropriate paddle or on the machine (depending on the model of defibrillator).

4 When the paddles are charged (indicated by a beeping sound), alert the cardiac arrest team that you are ready to defibrillate the patient. Ensure that no one is in contact with the patient's bed and that the floor is dry underneath the feet of the operator, as the bed and a wet floor conduct electrical currents. Press the paddles firm and flat against the patient's chest wall. 'One paddle is placed on the mid-axillary line over the sixth left intercostal space and the other is placed on the right parasternal area over the second intercostal space' (see Figure 5.8; ARC 1993, p 618). The paddles are placed in this position so that, as the current moves from one paddle to the other, it will pass through the heart.

5 Post defibrillation evaluate the patient's cardiac rhythm and monitor vital signs. Subsequent defibrillation using higher joules may be required if the patient's cardiac rhythm fails to revert to normal sinus rhythm or a more stable rhythm.

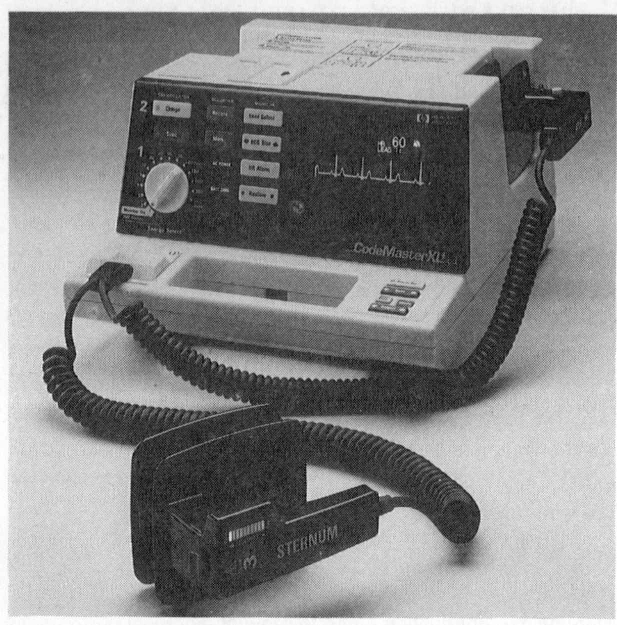

FIGURE 5.7 *Defibrillator (HP Code Master XL)*
Source Hewlett Packard

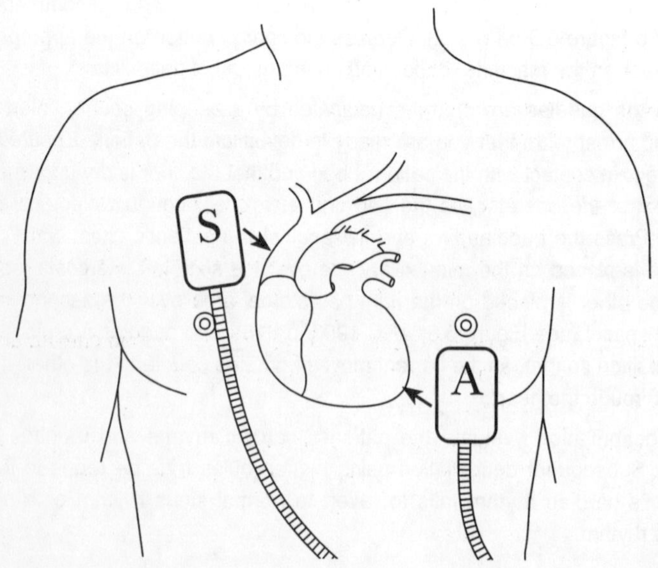

FIGURE 5.8 *Position of paddles during defibrillation (A = apex; S = sternum)*

CARDIOVERSION

Cardioversion is an electrical procedure used to correct abnormal cardiac rhythms, such as atrial flutter or atrial fibrillation, using a synchronised DC shock to create a more stable rhythm (preferably sinus rhythm; Camm & Ward 1993, pp 442–5). Synchronised means that the electrical energy required to terminate the arrhythmia is timed so that it coincides with the R wave. This is achieved by attaching the patient to the defibrillator's cardiac monitor. A switch on the defibrillator labelled 'synch' should be selected, together with the required amount of energy (75–100 joules). On the ECG screen you will notice vertical lines appearing above the QRS complex — this is the sensing spike from the defibrillator. The paddles are then positioned on the patient's chest and the discharge button is pressed. The defibrillator ensures that the charge is delivered to the nearest R wave. This reduces the risk of striking the top of the T wave. Position of the paddles for cardioversion is the same as for defibrillation (see Figure 5.8).

Care for patients undergoing cardioversion is the same as for defibrillation, except that a consent form is required from the patient before cardioversion can be performed. The patient also needs to be fasted before the procedure. All emergency resuscitation equipment is brought to the bedside and an anaesthetist should be in attendance until the procedure is finished. The patient is given a premedication, such as diazepam (valium), followed by a short-acting general anaesthetic agent, such as epontal.

It is possible that the rhythm may not revert to normal sinus rhythm, so a second charge may have to be delivered at higher joules.

IMPLANTABLE DEVICES

The development of reliable implantable devices has added new dimensions to the management of patients with malignant ventricular arrhythmias and patients with a high risk of cardiac arrest. The automatic implantable cardioverter/defibrillator (AICD) is a 'device designed to be implanted in the body which is capable of delivering cardioversion/defibrillation shocks of sufficient energy to the heart for the purpose of allowing the normal rhythm to be restored' (Asia/Pacific Medical Telectronics 1991). The AICD is best used in the following individuals:

- individuals who have survived at least one episode of sudden cardiac arrest resulting from ventricular tachycardia or ventricular fibrillation, and where an MI was not the precipitating cause
- individuals who have continued to experience recurrent episodes of life-threatening arrhythmias, despite pharmacological intervention (Buchok & Hardy 1991, p 1).

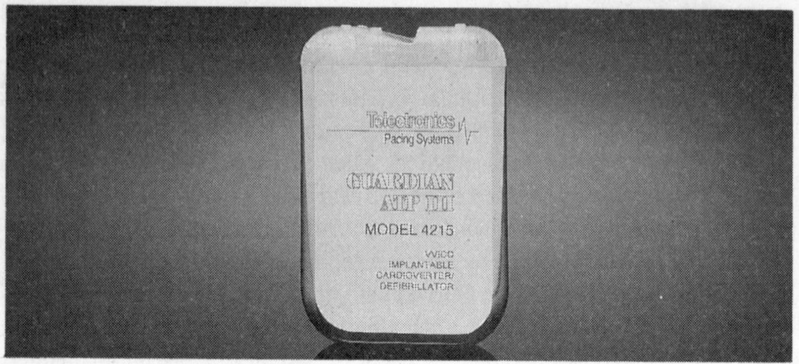

FIGURE 5.9 *Implantable cardioverter/defibrillator*

Source Asia/Pacific Medical Telectronics Pty Ltd

The AICD can be implanted using one of three methods.

- The *median sternotomy* approach is used when the patient is undergoing cardiac surgery. The defibrillation and the sensing/pacing electrodes are positioned on the epicardium and connected to the pulse generator. The pulse generator is placed in the abdomen (Buchok & Hardy 1991, p 2).
- Using the *left lateral thoracotomy* approach, the defibrillation patches are applied to the heart and the endocardial pacing/sensing electrode is positioned in the right ventricle via the left subclavian vein. The pulse generator is placed in the abdomen (Buchok & Hardy 1991, p 3).
- Implanting the AICD *transvenously* involves inserting the pacing/sensing leads and the defibrillator leads (transvenously) via the left subclavian vein. Depending ont he make and model of the AICD, one defibrillator electrode is placed in the right atrium and the other electrode is positioned in the apex of the right ventricle. The defibrillation patch is placed submuscularly in the anterior auxiliary line via a subcutaneous chest incision. This allows for the patch to be held in place more firmly (Buchok & Hardy 1991, p 4).

Electrophysical studies are undertaken on the patient in the operating theatre to ensure that the AICD is able to sense and terminate a malignant arrhythmia, such as ventricular fibrillation. Once the settings have been decided, these are programmed into the AICD's computer and the pulse generator is implanted in the abdomen.

Ventricular tachycardia is treated by antitachycardia pacing, cardioversion or defibrillation. Some AICDs also offer a bradycardia pacing feature (Buchok & Hardy 1991, p 1).

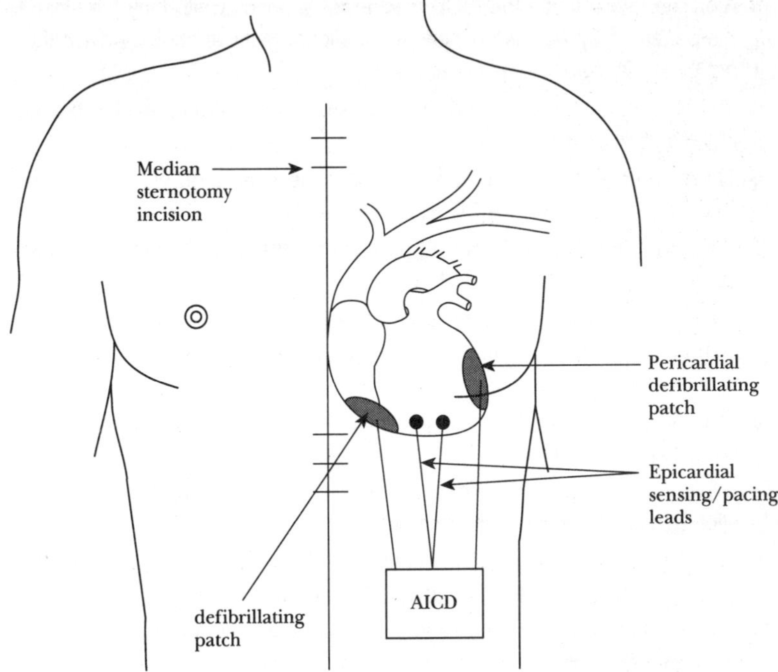

Figure 5.10 Position of the automatic implantable cardioverter/defibrillator (sternotomy approach)

Preparing the patient and family is very important prior to implanting the AICD. Relieve patient's anxiety by answering all questions, explaining briefly and simply about the procedure, emphasising postoperative care and discharge plans.

Postoperatively, the patient is admitted to the CCU for close observation and for monitoring the effectiveness of the implanted electrical device. Prevention of complications such as infection, bleeding and dislodgement or perforation of the leads, although seldom, must be maintained (Camm & Ward 1993, pp 442–5).

Specific postoperative care and discharge plan are as follows (Smeltzer & Bare 1992, pp 678–80).

1 Explain to the patient that the shock from the AICD, although painless, may feel like a blow to the chest.

2 When patient feels the shock they are advised to rest. The doctor must then be called. If the patient becomes unconscious, a member of the family must begin CPR and an ambulance must be called. If external defibrillation is needed, the paddles are positioned on the antero-posterior aspects of the thorax.

3 Alert the family that if the AICD discharges a shock while they are close to the patient, they will also experience a slight electrical shock. Advise them not to be alarmed, as it is not harmful.

4 The patient must carry a medical alert card or wear a medical alert bracelet in case of any emergency.

5 The patient must keep a diary recording the events of, when and under what circumstances the AICD discharges a shock.

6 Encourage family members and partners to attend and learn CPR procedures.

7 Advise the patient to avoid strong magnetic fields, such as radio and television transmitters or airport terminal security checks, as these may interfere with the AICD.

8 Emphasise the importance of continuously taking antiarrhythmic medications as prescribed.

9 Explain to the patient that during antitachycardia pacing, they may feel a slight fluttering sensation in the heart.

10 Ask the patient to advise their dentist and doctor of the AICD treatment — treatment they give the patient may alter functions of the AICD.

11 Encourage follow-up visits — it is during these visits that the AICD is reprogrammed according to the patient's needs.

CARDIAC PACING

Artificial cardiac pacemakers are electromechanical devices that are used to provide the heart with an electrical stimulus when the heart's natural pacemaker or conduction system fails to maintain an adequate cardiac output. Indications for inserting a pacemaker include:

- ventricular bradyarrhythmias which cause a reduction in cardiac output
- sinus arrest
- sick sinus syndrome to control the bradycardia or to treat the tacharrhythmia without causing irritation to the bradyarrhythmias
- transient arrhythmias following an MI, such as third degree AV block
- a precautionary measure before inserting a permanent pacemaker
- a precautionary measure following cardiac surgery
- symptomatic second degree and third degree AV block
- treatment of persistent tachyarrhythmias, for example ventricular tachycardia can be suppressed by putting the artificial pacemaker into overdrive
- significant periods of ventricular standstill
- bifascicular or trifascicular AV block
- during electrophysiological studies.

PACEMAKER COMPONENTS

Artificial pacemakers are comprised of two components: the pulse generator and the pacing catheter or lead wire.

The pulse generator

The pulse generator provides the energy required to transmit an electrical impulse and back up the sophisticated circuitry. A permanent pacemaker is comprised of a lithium battery which has a lifespan of between seven and ten years. The electrical system is capable of sending out timed signals and sensing cardiac activity, but unlike the AICD, cannot store information.

A temporary unit is used to pace people for a short time only. Its power is derived from a 9 V battery. Its ability to sense and trace is controlled externally by three dials. The *rate control dial* determines the rate at which the impulses are delivered from the pulse generator to the heart. The rate can be adjusted from between 30 and 180 pulses per minute (ppm). The *output dial* is used to adjust the amount of current required to elicit ventricular depolarisation. This is measured in milliampres (mA) and can be set between 0.1 and 20 mA. The *sensitivity dial* is the voltage required to respond to the heart's electrical activity and is measured in millivolts (mV). An 'on/off' switch has been designed so that the unit can be turned on easily, but to switch the unit off requires some manual dexterity! A battery test light indicates whether the pacing unit has sufficient power to operate efficiently.

The pacing catheter or leadwire

The pacing catheter (or leadwire) delivers an electrical impulse from the pulse generator through the insulating pacing catheter and electrode tip to the heart muscle. In the *unipolar* (one) electrode system the electrode has a negative polarity and the pulse generator is the positive electrode. Tall pacemaker spikes will be visible on the cardiac trace because the poles are situated apart from each other and the current is required to travel a large distance. In the *bipolar* (two) electrode system, one electrode is situated in the tip of the pacing catheter and has a negative polarity and the other, placed a few millimetres away (and proximal to the tip), assumes a positive polarity. Because the current only has to travel a short distance between the two electrodes, small pacing spikes will be visible on the cardiac trace (Nelson 1993, pp 193–7; Hudak, Gallo & Benz 1986, pp 145–6).

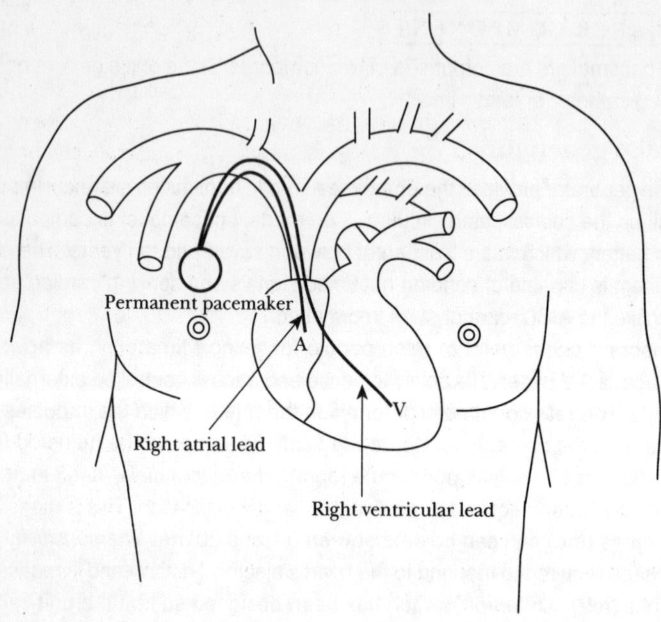

FIGURE 5.11 *Placement of a permanent pacemaker*

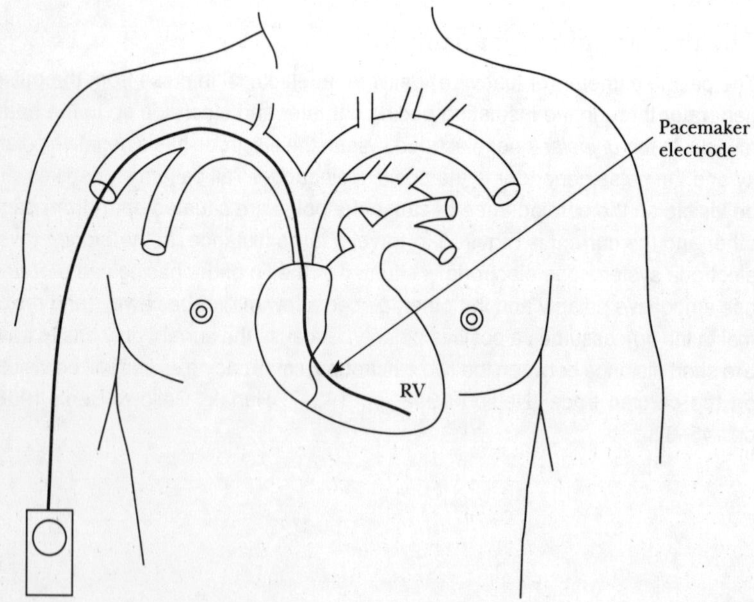

FIGURE 5.12 *Placement of a temporary pacemaker*

Placement of pacing leads

There are three techniques used for the placement of pacing leads. The *transmediastinal* technique is used during cardiac surgery. An electrode is implanted with a corkscrew tip into the epicardial surface of the left ventricle. A tunnel through the skin is created to allow the catheter (or leadwire) to be connected to an external pulse generator. When not in use, the catheter (or leadwire) is protected by a dry dressing.

Transvenous placement of the pacing wire is the most common placement procedure. Sites include the subclavian vein, jugular vein, femoral vein and antecubital fossa. The catheter (or leadwire) is inserted percutaneously or by using the 'cut-down' method to expose the vein. With the aid of an image intensifier, the pacing catheter is advanced to the apex of the right ventricle.

Transcutaneous pacing is a non-invasive form of pacing. Two pacing electrodes are attached to a pad applied to the patient's skin. One electrode marked 'back' is applied to the left side of the back just below the scapula and the other electrode marked 'front' is applied to the left side of the precordium. The pacing electrodes are changed every 24 hours or when necessary; the pacing electrodes come away easily and can render the pacing function inadequate (Appel-Hardin & Dente-Cassidy 1991, p 60).

PACEMAKER CLASSIFICATIONS

There are four pacing modes: fixed rate pacing, demand pacing, synchronous pacing and bifocal or AV sequential pacing or dual chamber pacing.

Fixed rate pacing (asynchronous)

Fixed rate pacing stimulates the heart to beat using a preset rate regardless of the heart's activity. For example, if patients were exercising, under normal circumstances the heart rate would increase to meet the physiological needs of the body. However, with a fixed rate pacemaker this does not occur. Today this mode of pacing is obsolete.

Demand pacing (synchronous)

In demand pacing the pacemaker contains a sensing mechanism which fires only on demand or when needed to stimulate atrial or ventricular contraction. Demand pacing is useful in the treatment of AV block, sinoatrial arrest and symptomatic bradyarrhythmias. The rate can be preset so that if the person's natural rate falls below the preset rate, the pacemaker discharges an impulse (Underhill et al 1989, p 770; Donovan 1990, p 9).

Bifocal or atrioventricular sequential pacing or dual chamber pacing

Bifocal pacing allows the atria and the ventricles to be paced sequentially. A sensing electrode is placed in the right ventricle. The right atrium and the right ventricle receive a pacing electrode; ventricular and atrial pacing depend on sensed ventricular activity. Once a ventricular event has been sensed, the atria and ventricle's pacing mode is inhibited. This type of pacing is useful in people experiencing sick sinus syndrome combined with degenerative disease of the ventricular conduction pathways (Donovan 1990, p 9; Underhill et al 1989, p 772). Other modes include atrial synchronised ventricular demand pacing and atrioventricular universal pacing.

PACEMAKER CODES

The American Heart Association and the American College of Cardiology adopted the British Pacing and Electrophysiology Group's (BPEG) suggested categories of pacemaker modes. The code uses three letters. The first two letters indicate which chambers of the heart are being paced and sensed: A = atria; V = ventricle; D = dual; O = none. The third letter of the code describes the mode of response to the sensed cardiac electrical potentials: I = inhibited (no firing of impulse when it senses electrical potentials); T = triggered (firing of an impulse every time it senses cardiac electrical potential); D = dual (both triggered and inhibited modes of response) and O = no sensing (no change in modes regardless of sensed cardiac electrical potential).

Code	Common designation	Comment
VOO — Paces the ventricle with no sensing	Fixed rate, asynchronous	Obsolete
VVI — Paces the ventricle, senses ventricular activity, ventricular impulses inhibit the pacemaker	Ventricular demand	Most commonly used in life-threatening bradycardia
AAI — Paces the atrium, senses atrial activity, atrial activity inhibits the pacemaker		Indicated in sinus bradycardia with normal AV conduction

cont next page

Code	Common designation	Comment
VAT — Paces the ventricle, senses atrial activity, atrial activity triggers ventricular pacing	Atrial synchronised, P wave triggered	Obsolete. Replaced by VDD and DDD
DVI — Paces both atrium and ventricle, senses only ventricular activity, ventricular activity inhibits atrial and ventricular pacing	AV sequential	Most commonly used dual chamber pacing mode in ICU
VDD — Paces the ventricle only, senses atrial and ventricular activity	Atrial synchronous, ventricular inhibited pacing	Indicated when normal sinus rhythm is present with a high degree AV block
DDD — Paces and senses both atrium and ventricle	AV universal	Often ideal but somewhat complicated

TABLE 5.1 *Pacemaker modes*

Source Donovan 1990, p 9

The three-letter identification pacemaker codes were adopted by the International Society Commission for Heart Disease for identifying functional capabilities of pacemakers. For example, **VOO** is described as asynchronous ventricular pacing, no adaptive rate control, and no antitachyarrhythmia functions. **DDD** is capable of pacing the atria and the ventricles (dual chamber), sensing both chambers, and response is inhibition in the atria with the occurrence of a sensed P wave and inhibition in the ventricles after a sensed R wave or VEB.

According to the BPEG, the main purpose for choosing a mode of pacing is to produce a feature of a normal sinus rhythm according to the following principles (Clark 1992, p 208):

- A = atrium paced/sensed unless contraindicated
- V = ventricles paced in the presence of actual or threatened atrioventricular blocks
- rate response may be used to overcome chronotropic incompetence.

Electrocardiograph features

Depending on which chamber is being paced, the ECG will record the pacing spikes on the following locations.

- Atrial pacing — pacing spikes will be seen followed by a P wave (Figure 5.13).

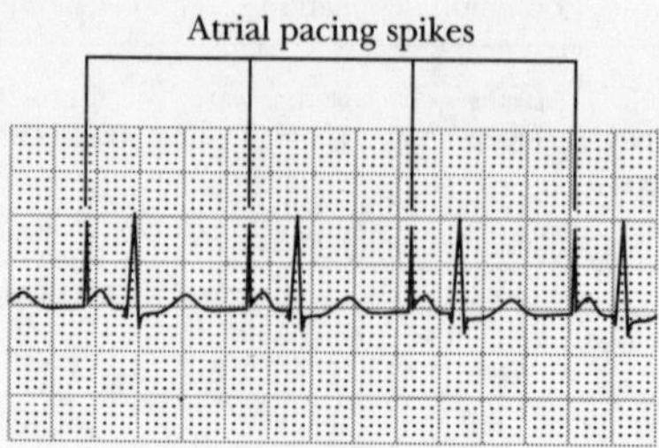

FIGURE 5.13 *Atrial pacing*

- Ventricular pacing — pacing spikes will be followed by a QRS complex (Figure 5.14).

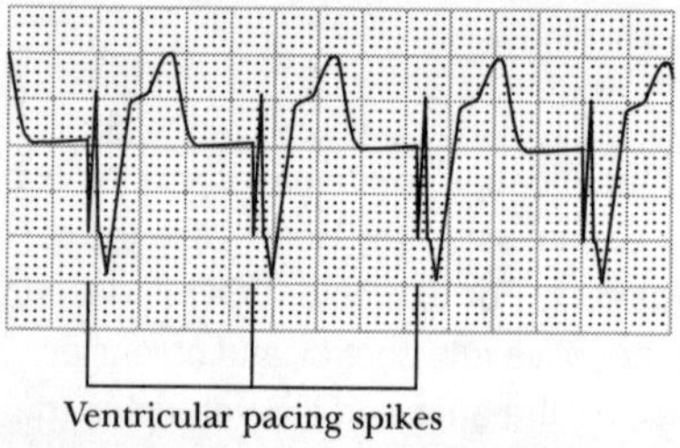

FIGURE 5.14 *Ventricular pacing*

- Dual chamber pacing — the P wave and the QRS complex are preceded by a pacing spike (Figure 5.15).

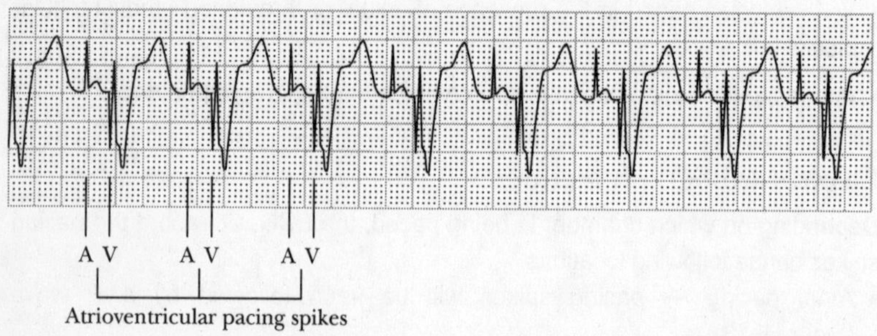

FIGURE 5.15 *Dual chamber pacing*

GENERAL PRINCIPLES IN THE CARE OF PATIENTS WITH TEMPORARY ARTIFICIAL PACEMAKERS

Many patients undergoing pacemaker insertion feel anxious about the procedure. Therefore, ensure that the patient and their significant others are given enough information to meet their needs. Initially, the procedure should be explained to them (including the risks involved) by their doctor. To ease the physical symptoms of anxiety, you may need to provide reassurance. Also encourage your patient to practise relaxation exercises.

The actual procedure may take place in a special room within the CCU or you may have to accompany your patient to the radiology department. If you are going to assist with the procedure, ensure that the patient is attached to a cardiac monitor, there is a sphygmomanometer to check the blood pressure, the emergency trolley is within easy reach and that all necessary equipment required to handle a cardiac arrest is present and in working order. A defibrillator should be included with the equipment.

During the procedure (performed under local anaesthetic) you need to assess the patient's condition continually. Observe their colour, assess whether they are restless and if they have chest pain. Record their vital signs at regular intervals and keep the medical staff informed. Check the patient's cardiac rhythm, especially while the pacing lead is being inserted into the heart, as there can be frequent ventricular ectopic beats caused by the lead irritating the ventricular walls (see Figure 5.12 on p 122). If there is multifocal ventricular ectopic beats or a short run of ventricular tachycardia is observed, notify the doctor immediately.

At the completion of the procedure the patient will be returned to the unit where they will remain monitored until the arrhythmia stabilises. Check that the pacemaker is functioning and that you can see a pacing spike on the cardiac trace. Ensure that the pulse generator is secured by either placing it in a cloth pouch and securing this to the patient's pyjama top or, in some units, that cotton tape is threaded through the sides of the pulse generator and it is suspended on an IV pole. Check that the pacing leads are securely connected to the terminals. The actual insertion site should be sealed with a clear occlusive dressing and regular observations should be made of the site for swelling, bleeding and redness. The site should be redressed according to unit protocol. Check the remainder of the limb distal and up to the insertion site for warmth, swelling, colour, sensation and movement. Report abnormalities and document your findings.

If the patient is confined to bed, ensure that they are encouraged to undertake passive and active limb exercises. Antiemboli stockings may be ordered, together with subcutaneous anticoagulant therapy.

There is a high risk of microshock in patients who have temporary pacemakers inserted. For this reason, critical care areas and high dependency wards have special electrical classifications to reduce the risk of microshock. Patients who have a pacemaker are normally placed in a class A electrical area. Ensure that the patient's bed is properly grounded and that any infusion pumps or other electrical equipment which is faulty is replaced. Staff should avoid leaning against electrical equipment while handling the patient. If there is an electrical fault, the current may pass through you to the patient and result in an arrhythmia. When handling pacemaker terminals it is a good idea to use rubber gloves. Encourage patients to use battery-operated shavers and transistor radios.

CARE OF PATIENTS WITH A PERMANENT PACEMAKER.

Preoperative care

Ensure that the patient has been fully briefed about the procedure and that a consent form has been signed by the patient and the doctor who witnessed the signature.

The patient is normally fasted six to eight hours before the operation if they are to have a general anaesthetic, or a few hours before a local anaesthetic. One hour before surgery the patient is given light sedation. The procedure is performed in the operating theatre by a cardiac surgeon using the aseptic technique. The pacing lead is inserted using an image intensifier to guide the pacing catheter to its position and the pulse generator box is inserted into the pectoral muscle just below the right or left clavicle, or is inserted into the abdomen.

Postoperative care

The patient's vital signs should be recorded at regular intervals until stable.

The patient should be attached to a cardiac monitor or a telemetry unit so that their rhythm can be observed to see whether the pacemaker is functioning correctly. Daily rhythm strips should be collected and filed in the patient's medical record.

Patients should be encouraged not to lie on their affected side, as this may lead to fracture of the pacing lead (see Figure 5.11 on p 122).

Possible pacemaker complications

After inserting a permanent pacemaker, the patient may experience extra cardiac stimulation in the form of pectoral muscle twitching or hiccoughs (especially in abdominally placed pulse generators). Decreasing the pacemaker voltage or the duration of the pacing pulse may alleviate this affect.

Failure for the pacemaker to capture is characterised on the ECG by no evidence of ventricular or atrial depolarisation after the pacing spike. The patient usually complains of unusual tiredness or lightheadedness. It can be caused by lead dislodgment, a flat battery or fractured pacing lead. It is best to replace the faulty parts.

Failure to pace is characterised on the ECG by the absence of any pacemaker activity. Patients may feel lightheaded, experience syncopal episodes and there may be hypotension or bradycardia. The problem is caused by fracture or displacement of the pacing lead or failure of the pulse generator (either the battery or the circuitry). It is best resolved by replacing the faulty parts.

Failure to sense is characterised on the ECG by the pacemaker spikes not appearing in their normal position. Instead, they appear in the ST segment or on the T wave. Failure to sense is dangerous because the spike may precipitate ventricular fibrillation. It is caused by lead dislodgement, electrolyte disturbances and scar tissue formation around the tip of the pacing lead, leading to an increased pacing threshold. The leads should be replaced or repositioned.

If the patient should require emergency defibrillation, the permanent pacemaker should be switched off with the aid of a magnet. Care should be taken not to place the paddles over the top of the pacemaker as it not only damages the unit, but myocardial damage may also result. If the patient has a temporary pacemaker, it should also be switched off prior to defibrillation.

It is important to encourage the patient to gently move the affected arm to prevent frozen shoulder syndrome. Patients may also be ordered subcutaneous anticoagulant therapy to prevent blood clots from forming around the pacing leads.

The suture line (and/or puncture site for temporary pacemakers) should be checked daily, observing for signs of infection, swelling and inflammation, and treated according to the unit's protocol. Prior to discharge for permanent pacemakers, a chest X-ray should be taken to ensure that the pacing lead is positioned correctly. The pacemaker function is also checked.

Following implantation of a permanent pacemaker, patient education should begin. This includes issues such as:

- checking own pulse rate daily for regularity, but more so for rate
- reporting for regular follow-ups
- consulting the doctor as soon as problems occur
- carrying an alert card at all times, especially when travelling, which includes information about settings of the pacemaker
- avoiding contact sports, such as football, as this could damage the pacemaker or cause lead fracture.

All pacemaker manufacturers provide patient education materials which you can refer to or give to the patient. Patients should also be made aware of local heart associations and the services they can provide.

REFERENCES

Advanced Life Support Committee of the Australian Resuscitation Council 1993, 'Adult advanced life support: The Australian Resuscitation Council Guidelines', *Medical Journal of Australia*, vol 159, no 9, pp 616–21

Appel-Hardin, S & Dente-Cassidy, A M 1991, 'How to use a non-invasive temporary pacemaker', *Nursing 91*, vol 21, no 5, pp 58–64

Asia/Pacific Medical Telectronics Pty Ltd 1991, You and Your AICD, patient information, Sydney

Atwood, S, Stanton, C & Storey, J 1992, *Introduction to Basic Cardiac Dysrhythmias*, Mosby, St Louis

Australian Resusciation Council 1988, *Cardiopulmonary Resuscitation*, Fergie Colour Printers, Brisbane

Bates, B 1991, *Guide to Physical Assessment and History Taking*, J B Lippincott Company, Philadelphia

Buchok, S & Hardy, J 1992, 'The implantable cardioverter defibrillator' (article courtesy of Troy Burke, Clinical Technical Manager, Asia/Pacific Medical Telectronics Pty Ltd)

Bullock, B L & Rosendahl, P P 1992, *Pathophysiology: Adaptations and Alterations in Function*, 3rd edn, J B Lippincott Company, Philadelphia

Camm, A J & Ward, D E 1993, 'Treatment of tachycardia: Cardioversion, defibrillation and pacemakers', *Medicine International*, vol 21, no 11, pp 442–5

Carrieri, V K, Lindsey, A M & West C M 1993, *Pathophysiological Phenomena in Nursing: Human Response to Illness*, 2nd edn, W B Saunders, Philadelphia

Clark, M 1992, 'Selection of Pacemaker Mode for the Management of Symptomatic Bradycardias', in Rowlands, D (ed), *Recent Advances in Cardiology*, Churchill Livingstone, London

Cooper, D K, Valladares, B K & Futterman, L C 1987, 'Care of patients with automatic implantable cardioverter-defibrillators: A guide for nurses', *Heart and Lung*, vol 16, pp 640–8

Donovan, K 1990, 'Cardiac Pacing', in Oh, T E (ed), *Intensive Care Manual*, 3rd edn, Butterworths, Sydney

Fuller, J & Schaller-Ayers, J 1994, *Health Assessment: A Nursing Approach*, J B Lippincott Company, Philadelphia

Garrett, A E & Adams, V 1986, *Pocket Handbook of Common Cardiac Arrhythmias: Recognition and Treatment*, J B Lippincott Company, Philadelphia

Guzzetta, C E & Dossey, B M 1992, *Cardiovascular Nursing: Holistic Practice*, Mosby, St Louis

Harrison, G A 1994 (unpublished), Contents of a letter — the precordial thump, St Vincent's Hospital, Sydney

Hudak, C, Gallo, B & Benz, J 1986, *Critical Care Nursing. A Holistic Approach*, 5th edn, J B Lippincott Company, Philadelphia

Huszar, R J 1988, *Basic Dysrhythmias: Interpretation and Management*, Mosby, St Louis

Ignatavicius, D D & Bayne, M V 1991, *Medical Surgical Nursing: A Nursing Process Approach*, W B Saunders, Philadelphia

Jarvis, C 1992, *Physical Examination and Health Assessment*, W B Saunders, Philadelphia

Kruiper, P A 1990, 'Automatic implantable cardioverter-defibrillator as a therapeutic modality for recurrent ventricular tachycardia: A case study', *Cardiovascular Nursing*, vol 5, pp 6–12

Lamb, J I & Carlson, V R 1986, *Handbook of Cardiovascular Nursing*, J B Lippincott Company, Philadelphia

Lewis, S M & Collier, I C 1992, *Medical–Surgical Nursing: Assessment and Management of Clinical Problems*, 2nd edn, Mosby, St Louis

Mandel, W J 1987, *Cardiac Arrhythmias: Their Mechanisms, Diagnosis and Management*, J B Lippincott Company, Philadelphia

Mirowski, M, Reid, P R, Mower, M M, Watkins, L, Gott, V L, Schauble, J F, Langer, A, Heilmann, M S, Kolenik, S A, Fischell, R E & Weisfelgt, M L 1986, 'Termination of malignant ventricular arrhythmias with an implantable automatic defibrillator in human beings', *New England Journal of Medicine*, vol 303, p 322

McCaffrey, M 1980, 'Understanding your patient's pain', *Nursing*, vol 10, p 26

Nelson, D 1993, 'Cardiac Pacemakers', in *Deciphering Difficult ECGs*, Springhouse Corporation, Springhouse

Norsen L, Telfair M & Wagner A 1986, 'Detecting Dysrhythmias', Springhouse Corporation, Springhouse, vol 16, no 11, pp 34–42

Platia, E V, Griffiths, L S C, Watkins, L, Mower, M M, Guarnieri, T, Mirowski, M & Reid, P R 1986, 'Treatment of malignant ventricular aneurysms with endocardial resection and implantation of the automatic cardioverter-defibrillator', *New England Journal of Medicine*, vol 314, p 312

Potter, P A 1990, *Pocket Guide to Physical Assessment*, Mosby, St Louis

Purcell, J & Burrows, S 1985, 'A pacemaker primer', *American Journal of Nursing*, vol 85, pp 553–68

Roth, L 1989, *Mosby's Drug Reference*, Mosby, St Louis

Scherer, J C 1992, *Introductory Clinical Pharmacology*, 4th edn, J B Lippincott Company, Philadelphia

Shaw, D B 1993, 'Pacemakers', *Medicine International*, vol 21, no 11, pp 453–56

Smeltzer, S & Bare, B 1992, *Brunner and Suddarth's Textbook of Medical and Surgical Nursing*, 7th edn, J B Lippincott Company, Philadelphia

Shoemaker, W C, Ayres, S, Grenvik, A, Holbrook, P R & Thompson, W L (eds) 1988, *Textbook of Critical Care*, W B Saunders, Philadelphia

Taylor, C, Lillis, C & LeMone, P 1989, *Fundamentals of Nursing: The Art and Science of Nursing Care*, J B Lippincott Company, Philadelphia

Thelan, L A, Davie, J K, Unden, L D & Lough, M E 1994, *Critical Care Nursing: Diagnosis and Management*, 2nd edn, Mosby, St Louis

Underhill, S L, Woods, S L, Froelicher, E S & Halpenny, C J 1989, *Cardiac Nursing*, 2nd edn, J B Lippincott Company, Philadelphia

Urden, L D, Davie, J K & Thelan, L A 1992, *Essentials of Critical Care Nursing*, Mosby, St Louis

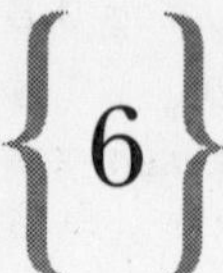

INTERPRETING A MYOCARDIAL INFARCTION FROM A 12 LEAD ECG

OBJECTIVES

After working through this chapter you should be able to:

- describe a normal 12 lead ECG
- describe and illustrate the characteristics of a normal Q wave, ST segment and T wave
- define the term myocardial infarction
- describe and discuss the ECG changes associated with a myocardial infarction
- state which ECG leads are affected according to the site of the myocardial infarction
- interpret a myocardial infarction from a 12 lead ECG

KEY WORDS

cardiac enzymes
infarction
injury
ischaemia
pathological Q waves
reciprocal changes
ST segment elevation
ST segment depression
subendocardial
T wave inversion
transmural

Before reading this chapter, you should revise the following topics.

Chapter 1—The location of the coronary arteries.

Chapter 2—The main purposes for recording a 12 lead ECG, electrode placement, normal wave progression and the appearance of a normal 12 lead ECG (see Figures 2.7 and 2.8 on pages 22 and 23 respectively).

This chapter discusses the ECG changes that occur following a myocardial infarction (MI) and the method used to interpret the 12 lead ECG. It is important to realise that other phenomena — the presence of a pulmonary embolism, chronic airways limiting disease — can also have an effect on the 12 lead ECG.

CASE STUDY

Jack Wilson is 52 years old, 172 cm tall and weighs about 95 kg. One Saturday afternoon while digging in the garden, Jack experiences an episode of severe retrosternal chest pain which radiates down the medial aspect of his left arm and up into his lower jaw. He also feels nauseous and is aware of his heart pounding in his chest. Jack calls out to his wife to ring for the ambulance. As he leans back against the fence, he recalls the similar episode of pain he experienced two days earlier. Only then, he thought it was just a bad case of indigestion.

On arrival in the emergency department of the hospital three-quarters of an hour later, Jack is still experiencing severe central chest pain, despite being given 5 mg IV morphine in the ambulance. He is pale and sweaty and has an overwhelming sense that something terrible is about to happen to him.

His observations are recorded: blood pressure, 145/95; heart rate is irregular at 110 bpm; his temperature is 36.8°C.

Jack is given an anginine tablet sublingually and oxygen via a Hudson's facemask at 8 L/min. He is given a further 5 mg morphine sulphate IV to help relieve his chest pain which hasn't settled since he was given the vasodilator. The RN explains to Jack that she will attach him to a cardiac monitor so that his heart rhythm can be monitored continuously. The rhythm observed is sinus tachycardia with an occasional ventricular ectopic beat. A full 12 lead ECG is recorded (see Figure 6.1) and the print-out is handed to you for interpretation.

The question you will probably ask yourself is 'Where do I begin?'

WHAT IS A MYOCARDIAL INFARCTION?

A myocardial infarction (MI) occurs when a coronary artery becomes occluded during a prolonged episode of myocardial ischaemia (angina). Failure of the oxygen-rich blood to reach that part of the myocardium causes irreversible damage and, as a consequence, myocardial death ensues. Damage to the myocardium may be limited to one layer of the muscle tissue or to the full thickness. Surrounding the necrotic or infarcted area is a zone of injury which, in turn, is surrounded by an ischaemic zone. The zones are not distinct entities, but have a tendency to overlap. In the days following the initial damage to the

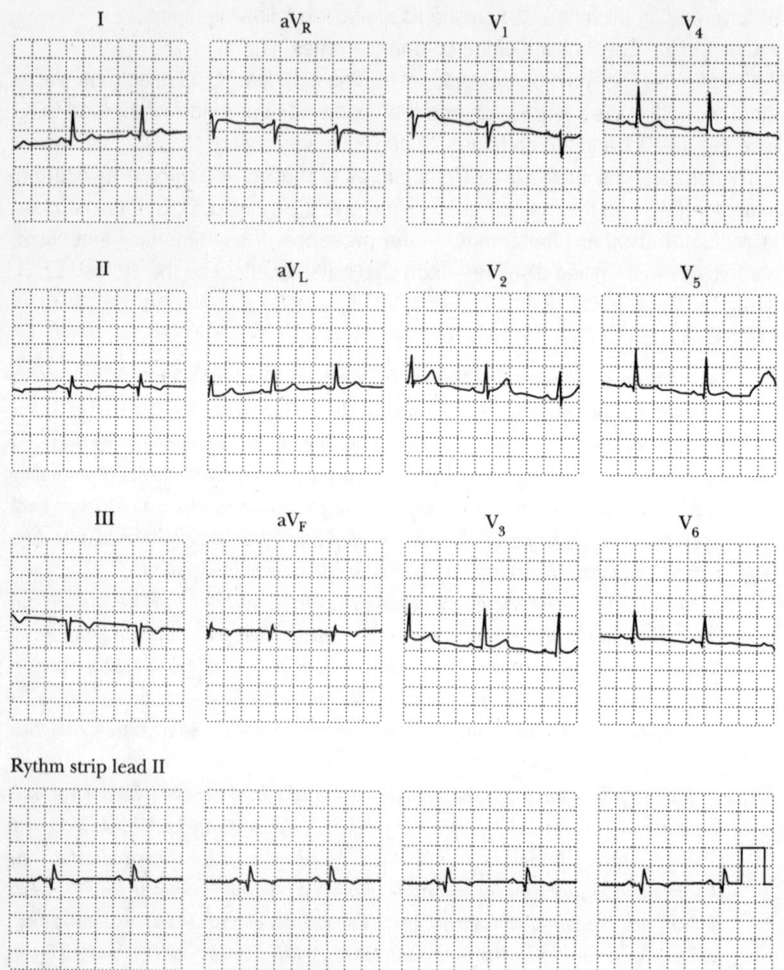

FIGURE 6.1 *Jack Wilson's 12 lead ECG*

myocardium, the zone of infarction may extend into the zones of injury and ischaemia because the tissue has been so badly affected and does not have the necessary blood supply available in order for the healing process to begin. For this reason it is very important that patients be admitted to a hospital within six hours of the infarction so that prompt treatment with either a vasodilator, such as glyceryl trinitrate (tridil), or an anti-thrombolytic agent, such as streptokinase or tissue plasminogen activator (TPA), can be administered to the patient intravenously. In doing so, there may not only be a chance of improving the blood supply to the affected area, but also a chance of limiting the size of the infarction.

AETIOLOGY OF CORONARY HEART DISEASE

Essentially, ischaemia can be the result of longstanding atherosclerosis in one or more of the coronary arteries. In this condition there is a build up of fatty, fibrous plaques that cause narrowing or an occlusion of an artery's lumen. Under these conditions it is not only the plaque which is responsible for occluding the vessel, but also the development of a clot or a thrombus.

The smooth muscle lining the inside of the coronary arteries has a tendency to develop sudden spasms, resulting in a decrease in the volume of blood reaching part of the myocardium. During severe episodes of coronary artery spasm, the blood flow may cease altogether to that part of the myocardium, resulting in tissue necrosis (Gibson 1990, p 30).

How do patients normally present?

Typically, the main symptom is severe central or retrosternal chest pain lasting more than half an hour. The pain tends to radiate to the medial aspect of the left arm, into the lower jaw and sometimes into the back between the scapulae. Patients often describe the pain as a sqeezing sensation or as if somebody has given them a bear hug. Associated signs and symptoms include nausea, vomiting, sweating, cold and clammy skin, restlessness, acute anxiety, a pounding or racing heart and a sense of impending doom. (Recall the case study at the beginning of this chapter.)

In comparison, some individuals experience very little, if any, pain.

HOW IS A MYOCARDIAL INFARCTION DIAGNOSED?

Chiefly, an MI can be diagnosed in three ways.

1 A thorough **clinical history** needs to be obtained from the patient. If the patient is not well enough, details can be collected from a relative. The details which the physicians need to know include: the site of the pain; precipitating factors, that is, what caused the pain or what activity was the patient undertaking when they first experienced the pain; and how long has the patient had the pain, that is, weeks, days, hours or is it the first attack? The doctor will want to know if there is a family history of heart disease and if any family members died as a result of heart disease. There is a familial tendency in heart disease (eg sudden death syndrome). The doctor will also want to know if the patient has had any previous admissions to hospital with chest pain and, if so, what the final diagnosis was.

   Central retrosternal chest pain is not always associated with the heart. In some circumstances it can be related to the intestinal tract (eg oesophagitis, indigestion) or the presence of gastric ulcers. On other occasions, central retrosternal chest pain can be related to respiratory conditions such as pleurisy, pneumonia, or the development of a pneumothorax (air in the pleural space).

The doctor will also want to know if and when the patient was given pain relief, the type and the route of administration, and its effectiveness.

2 A series of **blood tests** will be undertaken, which include electrolyte levels, a full blood count and measurement of the cardiac enzymes (creatnine kinase (CK), aspartate transaminase (AST) and lactic dehydrogenase (LDH)). Creatnine kinase has an isoenzyme that is specific to cardiac muscle which is important, especially if patients have been given intramuscular injections or have been defibrillated. During these procedures, CK is released from the damaged striated muscle tissue into the serum. If the enzyme was measured without this information, the CK result would be considerably higher than expected, indicating that the patient had suffered a massive MI. In order to know the proportion of cardiac muscle which has been affected, the doctor will ask for a CKMB to be measured. MB represents the isoenzyme for heart muscle.

The CKMB measurement indicates the extent of the infarction. For example, a measurement of 300 may indicate that the patient has had a small myocardial infarction (or perhaps a subendocardial infarction), whereas a reading of 2000 may indicate that the patient has sustained extensive damage to the myocardium.

Blood samples to measure CK should be collected on admission and then six-hourly, as the maximum level of the enzyme occurs between six and 12 hours following the MI, returning to near normal levels after 24 hours.

Lactic dehydrogenase usually begins to appear in the plasma within 24 hours after the onset of the myocardial infarction and as a rule does not reach its peak level until 24–36 hours later. It can remain elevated for at least a week before returning to its normal level, which is an advantage for people who present to hospital late with a suspected myocardial infarction and in whom the CK has long since returned to its normal level.

Aspartate transaminase tends to peak within five hours following an MI and gradually subsides, returning to normal levels after five days.

The normal levels for each of the cardiac enzymes are:

CK	0–230 U/L
CKMB, straight rate	0–6%
CKMB	0–2.2%
LDH	100–190 U/L
AST	0–37 U/L

Source Northern Area Health Service, Sydney

3 A **full 12 lead ECG** recorded over at least three consecutive days assists in confirming the diagnosis of an MI. The wave patterns reveal where infarction has occurred in the myocardium and also indicates the presence of myocardial injury and ischaemia.

ELECTROCARDIOGRAPHIC CHANGES FOLLOWING AN ACUTE MYOCARDIAL INFARCTION

Electrocardiographic changes following an acute MI are as follows.

1 A **pathological Q wave** is indicative of myocardial necrosis and may appear on the ECG within a few hours of the infarction occurring, or it may gradually develop over a few days. Electrically, infarcted tissue does not transmit impulses, therefore a positive electrode positioned over the affected site records a wide negative deflection. The electrical impulse is reflected off the damaged cells causing a QS wave to be seen in the affected leads.

QS waves are normal occurrences in leads aV_R, V_1, and sometimes in leads III and V_2, and usually have nothing to do with MIs (unless, of course, there are other signs on the ECG indicating that myocardial injury has taken place). Unlike the appearance of a normal Q wave, a pathological Q wave should be at least one-third the height of the R wave and greater than 0.04 seconds in duration (see Figure 6.2). Pathological Q waves also remain on the ECG for many years as a telltale reminder of the patient's past history. Some patients who have undergone a 12 lead ECG are very surprised when they are informed by their physician that they have had a previous MI. Many patients recall a time when they experienced a severe episode of chest pain, but thought it was indigestion or caused by something they were doing at that moment.

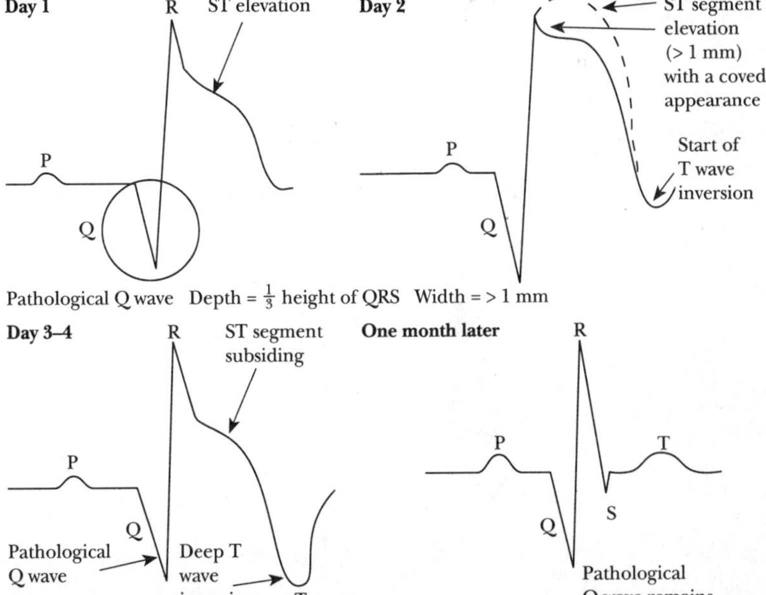

FIGURE 6.2 *ECG changes occurring with a myocardial infarction*

Source Adapted from McRae 1983, p 206

A pathological Q wave is seen only if the patient has had what is termed a *full thickness infarction* (ie from the endocardium to the epicardium). The term originally used to describe this type of infarction was *transmural*, but this has recently been replaced by the term *Q-wave* infarction. In patients who have experienced subendocardial infarctions, there is no pathological Q wave and hence the term *non-Q-wave* infarction is applied (Romanini 1994, p 174).

2 **ST segment elevation** indicates that there has been injury to the myocardium (see Figure 6.2). The segment should be elevated at least 1 mm in height to be of significance. In some traces it can be as high as 10 mm. The elevated portion of the ST segment has a convex or a coved appearance. Normally, elevated ST segments are present from the onset of the infarction and are seen in the leads positioned over the affected area. In the leads opposite the site of the infarction, the ST segment takes on a depressed appearance, and is termed a *reciprocal change* (see Figure 6.3). Therefore, when reading a report of the patient's 12 lead ECG, it may say 'ST elevation in leads V_1–V_4 with reciprocal changes in leads II, III and aV_F'.

From the second or third day following the MI, the ST segment begins to return to the baseline and within four weeks assumes its normal position. ST elevation is thought to occur because the inside of the injured cell becomes

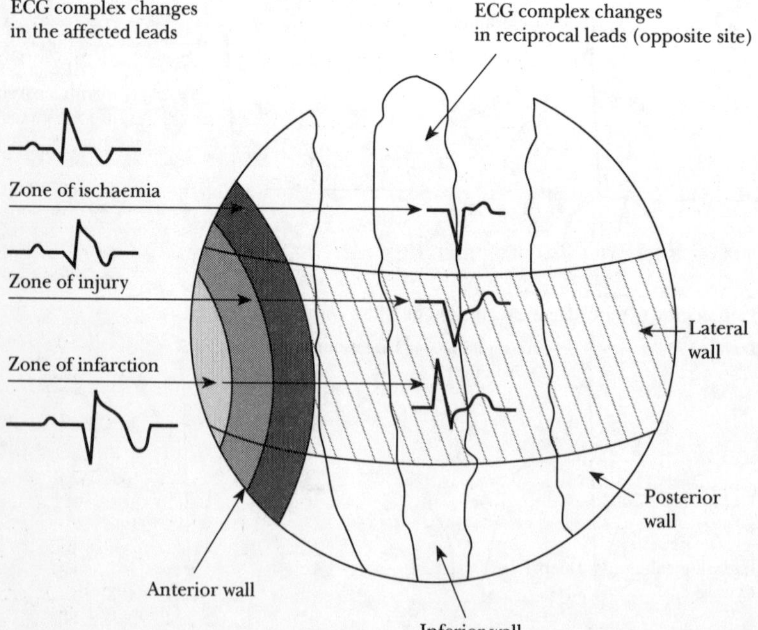

FIGURE 6.3 *Reciprocal ECG changes following a myocardial infarction*

more positive (to about –20 mV). An electrode placed over the injured site and facing the direction of the positive wave of electrical movement through the heart yields an elevated ST segment on the ECG.

3 Myocardial ischaemia is represented by **T wave inversion**. The T wave is symmetrically inverted. Sometimes it may only be slightly inverted to a depth of 1–2 mm or may be up to a depth of 8 mm. The T wave may be seen on the ECG from day one of the MI, but usually starts to appear by day two, and gradually deepens as the MI evolves. It may also become a permanent feature on the ECG, but normally it resumes its upright position after a couple of months.

The rate at which the patient recovers from the MI is largely dependent upon the extent of the damage and the actual site of the MI in the ventricular walls. Most MIs involve the left ventricle; affecting either the anterior, inferior, lateral or posterior walls. An MI can involve the right ventricle, but this is not as common, due to the fact that the left ventricle is so much larger and because there is a greater blood supply, which involves three of the major coronary arteries.

The site of the MI may not be confined to just one area and may overlap into other parts of the ventricular wall. Therefore, an MI occurring in the anterior wall of the ventricle may involve the lateral aspect or the septum, in which case the MI is referred to as an *anterior lateral* MI or an *anteroseptal* MI respectively. Similar phenomena occur with the inferior, lateral and posterior sites.

Whatever the site, the ECG changes will be seen in those leads overlying the affected area. Table 6.1 summarises the sites of the MI, the leads involved, the coronary artery affected by the occlusion, the structures of the heart which are affected as a result of the MI, and the complications that the patient may develop as a result of this type of MI.

Site of myocardial infarction	Leads	Part of heart affected	Occluded coronary artery	Complications
Anterior	V_1–V_3; reciprocal changes in LII, LIII, aV_F.	Blood supply to AV node; apex of left ventricle; anterior left ventricle; anterior two-thirds of left ventricle; two-thirds of interventricular septum	Left anterior descending artery	Arrhythmias: VEB, VT, VF; AV blocks: first degree, second degree, third degree
Extensive anterior	V_1–V_6, LI, aV_L; reciprocal changes in LII, LIII, aV_F	As above	Left main coronary artery, left anterior descending artery, circumflex artery	Left ventricular aneurysm; cardiogenic shock; papillary muscle rupture; CCF; rupture of the left ventricle; VF; VT

cont next page

Site of myocardial infarction	Leads	Part of heart affected	Occluded coronary artery	Complications
Anterior/ lateral	V_1–V_3, V_5, V_6, LI, aV_L	As for anterior MI	Left anterior descending artery; sometimes the circumflex artery	As for extensive anterior MI
Anterior/ septal	L_1, V_1–V_4	As above	Left main coronary artery; left anterior descending artery	As for anterior MI
Inferior	LII, LIII, aV_F; reciprocal changes in LI, aV_L	Blood supply to SA node and AV node; right atrium; posterior portion of left ventricle; diaphragmatic surface of left ventricle; right ventricle	Right coronary artery	Arrhythmias: AEB, atrial fibrillation, atrial flutter; conduction defects; AV blocks: first degree, second degree, third degree
Inferior/ lateral	LII, LIII, aV_F, aV_L, LI, V_5, V_6	As above	As above; circumflex artery	As above
Septal	V_1–V_4	As above	Left main coronary artery; left anterior descending artery	Rupture of the interventricular septum; formation of atrial or ventricular septal defect
Lateral	LI, aV_L, V_5, V_6; reciprocal changes in LII, LIII, aV_F, V_1	Lateral aspect of left ventricular wall; apex of the heart	Circumflex artery; left main coronary artery	Arrhythmias: VEB; rupture of left ventricle; formation of left ventricular aneurysm
Posterior	Tall, broad R waves; ST depression in V_1 and V_2; reciprocal changes (ST elevation) in LII, LIII, aV_F	Left atrium; entire posterior wall of the heart; posterior one-third of interventricular septum	Either the circumflex branch of the left coronary artery or an occlusion in the right coronary artery	Right ventricular failure; arrhythmias: second degree AV block (Wenckebach)
Right ventricular	LII, LIII, aV_F	As for inferior/ lateral MI	Occlusion of right coronary artery	Arrhythmias: second degree AV block

TABLE 6.2 *Myocardial infarction sites*

Following an MI, one of the most common complications is the development of arrhythmias. To assist in assessing which patients may be at more risk of developing an arrhythmia, a special type of ECG can be utilised, that is, a signal-averaged ECG or SAECG. This test is capable of detecting conduction abnormalities that often precede life-threatening arrhythmias, such as ventricular tachycardia. The ECG can be performed at the patient's bedside by attaching six electrodes: five electrodes to the front of the patient's chest and one electrode on the patient's back. On the anterior chest wall, electrodes are located at the top of the sternum in the standard V_2 and the V_3 position, at the fourth intercostal space in the left mid-axillary line, one at the fourth intercostal space at the right mid-axillary line, and the ground electrode is placed at the right side of the eighth rib. On the posterior chest wall, one electrode is placed directly opposite the standard V_2 position on the anterior chest wall. This ECG detects repolarisation delays

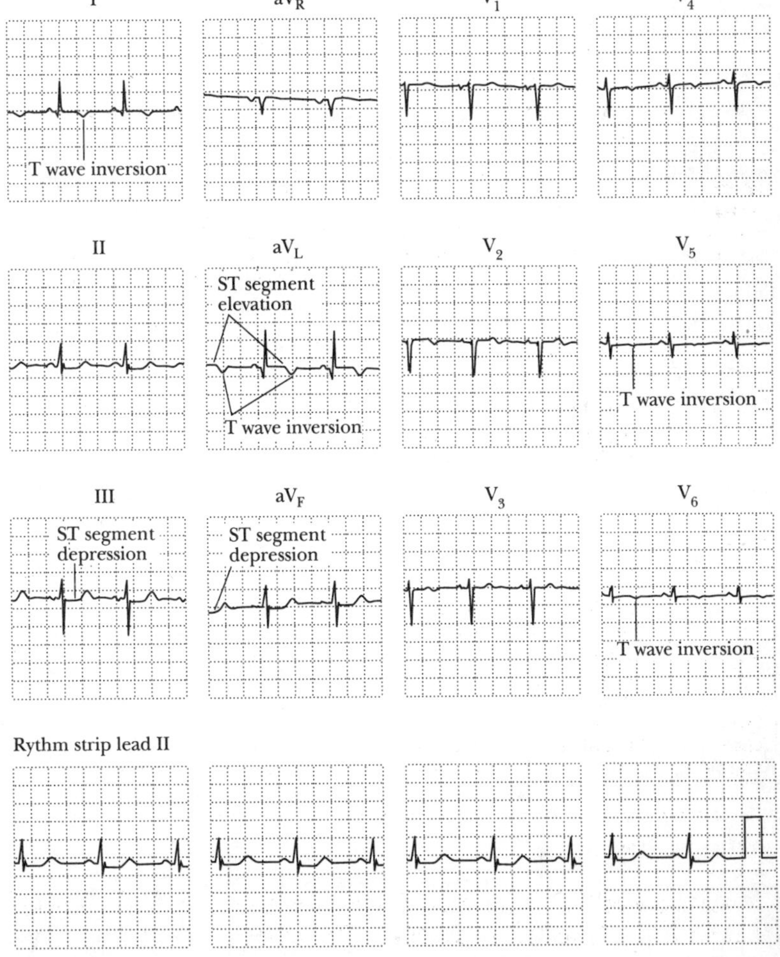

FIGURE 6.4 *12 lead ECG indicating evidence of an inferior subendocardial myocardial infarction with lateral ischaemia*

that occur when ischaemic or infarcted tissue impedes the flow of electrical impulses through the affected part of the myocardium, and which give rise to the discharge of ectopic beats, resulting in arrhythmias such as ventricular tachycardia (Murva 1993, pp 50–1). Currently, the SAECG is undergoing clinical trials in some major Sydney hospitals.

Figure 6.4 on page 141 shows a T wave inversion in the lateral leads, LI, aV_L, V_5 and V_6; ST segment depression in the inferior leads: LII, LIII, aV_F. The patient has probably had an inferior subendocardial MI with lateral ischaemia.

In Figure 6.5 there is widespread ST elevation in the anterior leads, V_1, V_2, V_3, V_4, V_5 and V_6 and slight elevation in LI. In aV_L there is the beginning of T wave

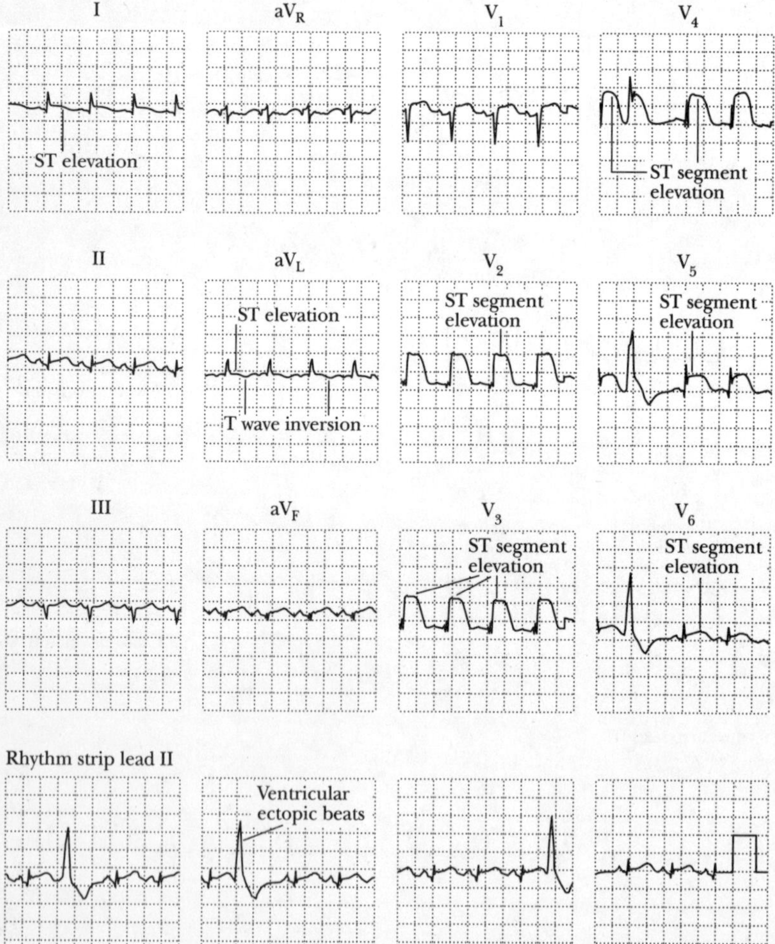

FIGURE 6.5 *12 lead ECG indicating evidence of an extensive anterior myocardial infarction*

inversion. There are ischaemic changes to the ST segment in the inferior leads, LII, LIII and aV_F. The patient has probably had an extensive anterior MI.

In Figure 6.6 there is ST segment elevation present in the inferior leads LII, LIII and aV_F, together with the beginning of T wave inversion. There are also pathological Q waves in LIII and aV_F. The Q waves in LII are too small to be of any significance. In the lateral leads there is ST segment depression in LI and aV_L, and in V_5 and V_6 there is ST segment flattening (ischaemic changes). The patient has probably had an inferior myocardial infarction with reciprocal changes in the lateral leads.

The 12 lead ECGs in Figures 6.4 and 6.7 indicate evidence of various MIs and myocardial ischaemias. (Note: the ECG recordings are one of a series from actual patients whose clinical history and cardiac enzyme results are unknown.)

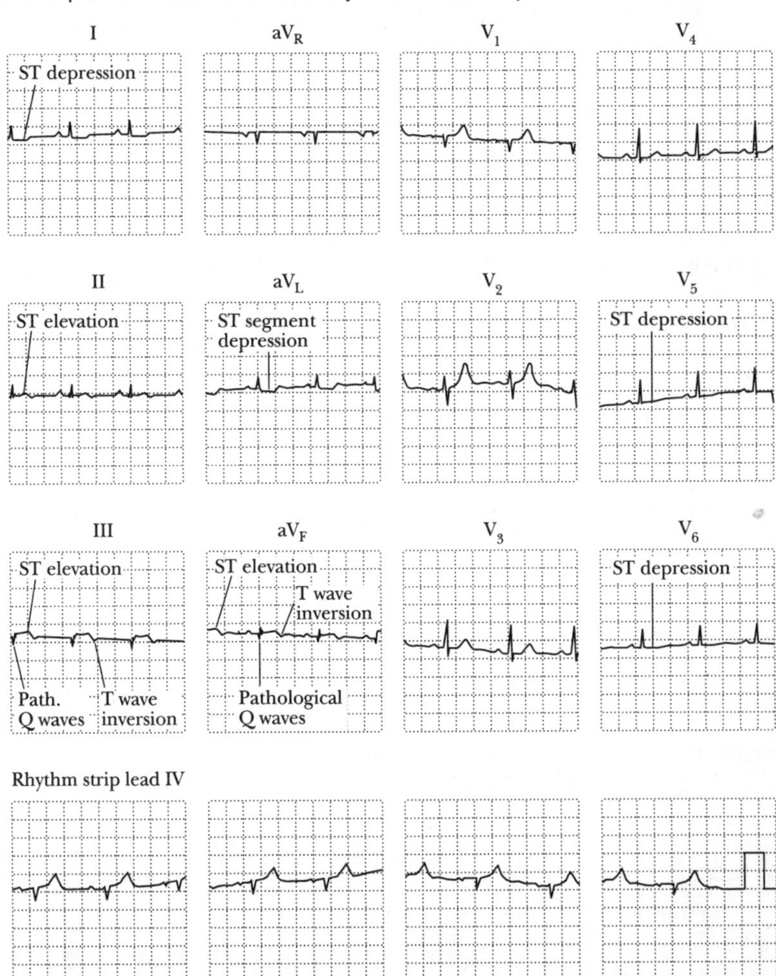

FIGURE 6.6 *12 lead ECG indicating evidence of an inferior myocardial infarction*

In Figure 6.7 there is ST segment elevation in LI, aV_L, V_2, V_3, V_4, V_5 and V_6. There is ST segment depression in the inferior (reciprocal) leads, LII, LIII and aV_F. There are pathological Q waves in V_2, V_3, V_4, V_5 and aV_L. It is probable that the patient has had an extensive anterior lateral myocardial infarction.

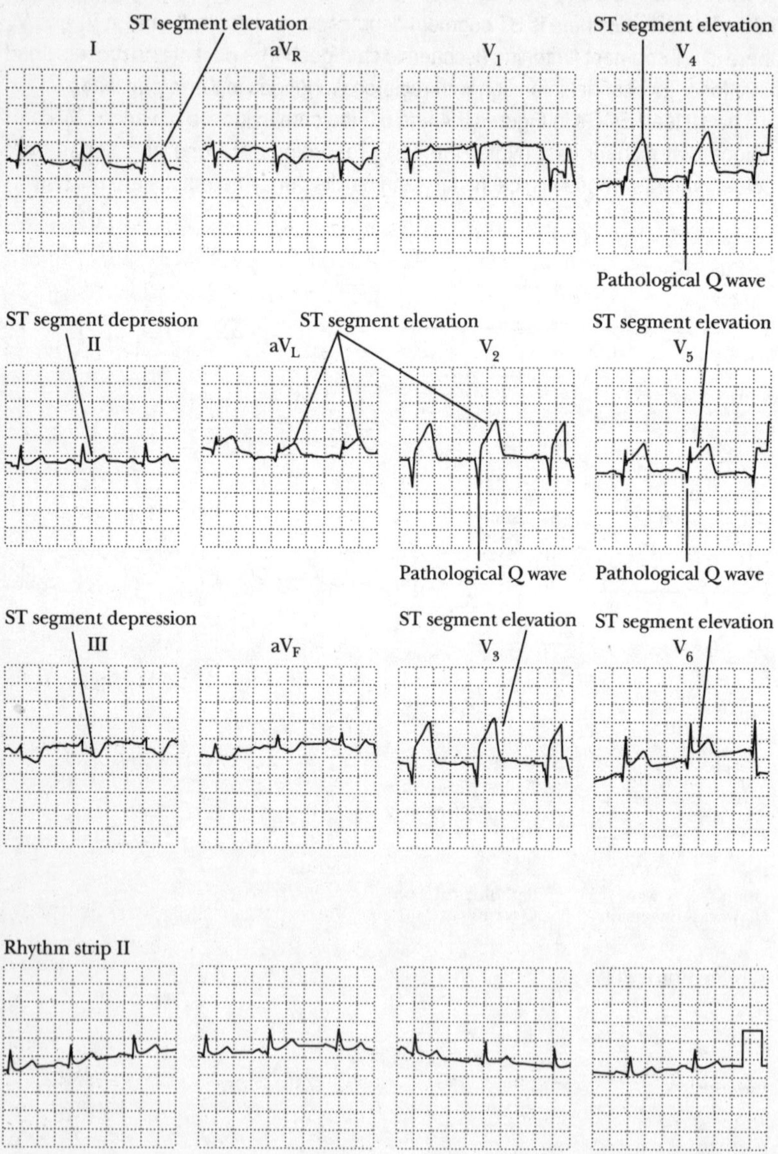

FIGURE 6.7 *12 lead ECG indicating evidence of an extensive anterior lateral myocardial infarction*

INTERPRETATION OF A MYOCARDIAL INFARCTION FROM A 12 LEAD ECG

As in arrhythmia interpretation, it is important to use a consistent method for interpreting the 12 lead ECG because essential information can be gained from this assessment tool. Practising this skill as much as possible benefits you *and* the patient.

There are seven steps used to interpret an MI from a 12 lead ECG.

STEP 1

Before examining the patient's trace, it is important to read their medical record and note their past health history. Have they previously suffered an MI as evidenced by a pathological Q wave on the latest trace? Note also the reasons for the patient's admission, and what type chest pain, if any, was experienced and the character of the pain. Read the pathology results and check that the cardiac enzyme levels are within the normal range. Knowing this information provides valuable clues while examining the 12 lead ECG and assists with subsequent management plans for the patient.

STEP 2

Examine the quality of the 12 lead ECG. Ensure that: (i) the ECG has been standardised to 1 mV by looking for the calibration mark on the printed record; (ii) a lead II cardiac rhythm has been recorded at the bottom of the page (this depends on the make and the model of the ECG machine — some automatically do, others do not record the rhythm); (iii) all the waves of the ECG complex can be seen clearly and that the QRS complex is within the confines of the graph paper; and (iv) all the leads have been recorded and there is normal wave progression in the V (chest) leads.

In particular, note lead aV_R — normally the QRS complex in this lead has a negative deflection. If it has a positive deflection, the limb electrodes may have been attached incorrectly and the 12 lead ECG will have to be repeated.

STEP 3

Examine each lead individually, noting any signs of an acute MI, such as ST elevation greater than 1 mm, pathological Q waves and T wave inversion. If present, note which leads are involved.

STEP 4

Look for reciprocal changes in the leads on the opposite side to the suspected infarction site. These changes may include ST segment depression. If these signs are present, note which leads are involved.

Depending on the patient's clinical history, look for signs consistent with a previous MI, such as pathological Q waves.

STEP 5

Compare the current findings with a 12 lead ECG recorded within the last 24 hours to see whether or not there is an evolving infarction pattern present. If this is the first 12 lead ECG recorded, make a note of your findings, together with the information from the patient's clinical history and the cardiac enzyme results.

STEP 6

Determine the site of the MI and interpret the 12 lead ECG.

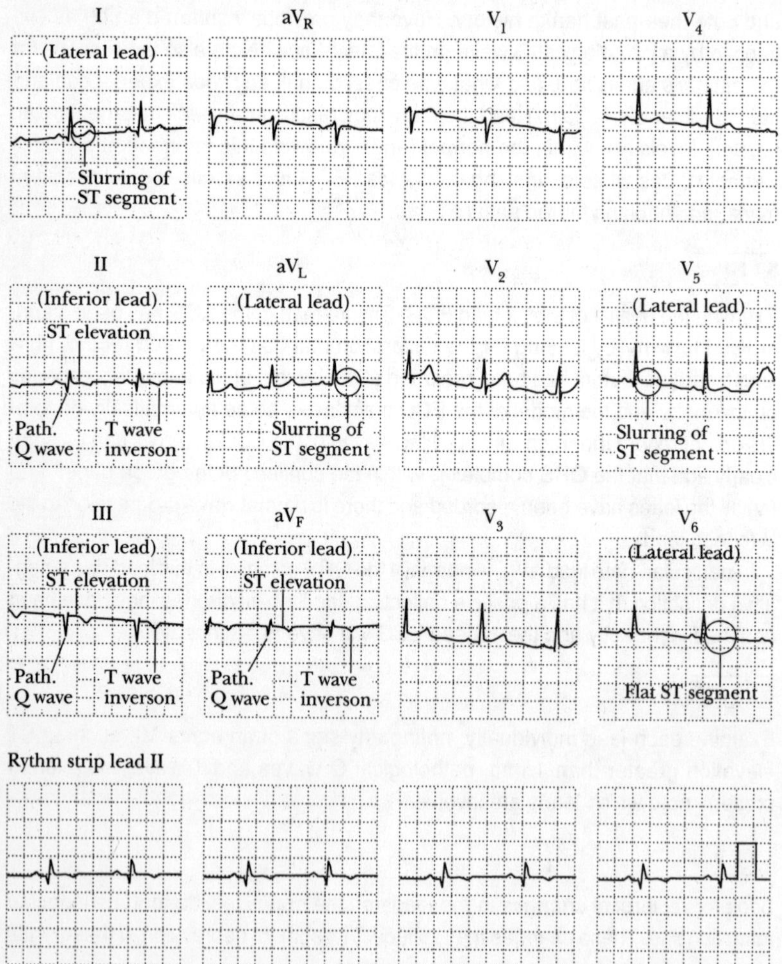

FIGURE 6.8 *Jack Wilson's 12 lead ECG*

STEP 7

Interpret the cardiac rhythm.

Now, using Jack Wilson's 12 lead ECG on page 146 we will apply these steps.

Step 1 All we know about Jack's past clinical history is that two days prior to his admission he experienced a similar episode of chest pain. The cardiac enzyme results are not available. Jack is overweight for his height and this is one of the recognised risk factors in cardiovascular disease.The pain and the fear that he feels about his life ending prematurely (dying before 70 years of age) is typical of the physical and mental symptoms associated with an MI.

Step 2 The ECG is a clear trace; all the leads have been recorded and the ECG has been standardised to 1 mV. A LII cardiac rhythm has been recorded at the bottom of the page.

Step 3 Examining the 12 lead ECG, there are pathological Q waves in LII, LIII and aV_F. In these same leads there is some ST segment elevation and T wave inversion is present.

Step 4 There are reciprocal changes (ischaemic) in the lateral leads. In V_6 the ST segment is flat and in the other lateral leads (V_5, LI and aV_L), there is a slurring of the ST segment.

Step 5 The pathological Q waves present are associated with the current problem.

Step 6 Jack has probably suffered an inferior MI and has reciprocal ischaemic changes in the lateral leads.

Step 7 Jack's cardiac rhythm is normal sinus rhythm. (The tachycardia noted initially may have been related to Jack's anxiety and his pain.)

In Chapter 7 there are six 12 lead ECGs for the reader to practise the skill of interpretation. Worked answers have been provided in Appendix 2.

REFERENCES

Australian Institute of Health and Welfare 1992, *Australia's Health 1992*, The Third Biennial Report of the Australian Institute of Health and Welfare, Australian Government Publishing Service, Canberra

Aragon, D & Martin, M 1993, 'What you should know about thrombolytic therapy for acute MI', *Australian Journal of Nursing,* vol 93, no 9, pp 24–31

Dubin, D 1978, *Rapid Interpretation of EKGs*, Cover Publishing Company, Tampa, Florida

Grant, C & Lapsley, H M 1993, *The Australian Health Care System 1992*, School of Health Services Management, University of New South Wales, Kensington

Gibson, R 1990, 'Myocardial Infarction', in *Patient Teaching Loose Leaf Library,* Springhouse Corporation, Springhouse

Guyton, A 1991, *Textbook of Medical Physiology,* 8th edn, W B Saunders with HBJ International, Philadelphia

Hudak, C, Gallo, B & Benz, J 1990, *Critical Care Nursing. A Holistic Approach*, J B Lippincott Company, Philadelphia

Hunt, D, Carlisle, C, Chan, W & Kertes, P 1983, *Coronary Care Workbook. A Handbook for Coronary Care Nurses*, 5th edn, Excerpta Medica, Amsterdam & Royal Melbourne Hospital, Melbourne

Holloway, N M 1993, *Nursing the Critically Ill Adult*, 4th edn, Addison-Wesley Publishing Company, Redwood City

Johnson, P 1993, 'Coronary heart disease in rural NSW: One country hospital's experience', *The Australian Journal of Rural Health*, vol 1, no 2, February, pp 19–23

Julian, D 1984, *Cardiology*, 4th edn, Balliere Tindall, London

Meltzer, L, Pinneo, R & Kithchell, J R 1983, *Intensive Coronary Care. A Manual for Nurses*, 4th edn, Robert J Brady Company, Bowie

Murva, J 1993, 'A closer look at the heart SAECG', *RN*, May, pp 50–3

National Heart Foundation of Australia 1992, *Heart Facts*, National Heart Foundation of Australia, Sydney

Parsons, C 1990, 'Cross-Cultural Issues in Health Care', in Reid, J & Tromph, P (eds), *The Health of Immigrant Australia*, Harcourt Brace Jovanovich, Sydney

Pepine, C J 1989, 'New concepts in the pathophysiology of acute myocardial infarction', *American Journal of Cardiology*, vol 64, 18 July, pp 2b–8b

Romanini, J & Daly, J (eds), 1994 *Critical Care Nursing. Australian Perspectives*, Harcourt Brace and Company, Sydney

Thompson, P L 1990, 'Myocardial Infarction', in Oh, T E (ed), *Intensive Care Manual,* Butterworths, Sydney

Underhill, S, Woods, S, Froelicher, E & Halpenny, C 1989, *Cardiac Nursing*, 2nd edn, J B Lippincott Company, Philadelphia

Wadsworth, L, Dragoo, C, Lapenna, S, Goodwin, S, Palabrica, D F & Hillard, S 1982, 'Intracoronary streptokinase infusion', *Nursing 82,* May, pp 58–65

Watters, R E, Johnson, G E, Hannah, K J & Zerr, S R 1994, *Pharmacology and the Nursing Process. The Australian Edition*, W B Saunders & Balliere Tindall, Sydney

Young, C M 1986, *Selection and Survival: Immigrant Mortality in Australia*, Australian Government Publishing Service, Canberra

{7}

EXERCISES IN CARDIAC RHYTHM AND 12 LEAD ECG INTERPRETATION

PART A — CARDIAC RHYTHM INTERPRETATION

HOW TO READ THE RHYTHM STRIPS

Analyse the cardiac rhythm strips in the following exercises using the method we introduced to you in Chapter 2. The paper speed is 25 mm/sec and the monitoring lead is LII.

1 Is the rhythm regular?

2 What is the heart rate?

3 Is there a P wave? What is its relationship to the QRS complex and the T wave? What is the shape of the P wave?

4 Calculate the PR interval. Does it fall within the normal time duration?

5 What is the shape of the QRS complex? Is it small or wide? Calculate the time duration of the QRS complex. Is it within normal limits?

6 Can you visualise the ST segment? Does it appear depressed or elevated? (Remember, an MI cannot be interpreted from a single monitoring lead. You will need to see a full 12 lead ECG.)

7 Is there a T wave? What is its shape? Does it follow the QRS complex?

8 Now, interpret the cardiac rhythm strip.

Answers to the exercises appear in Appendix 2.

EXERCISES

Exercise 1

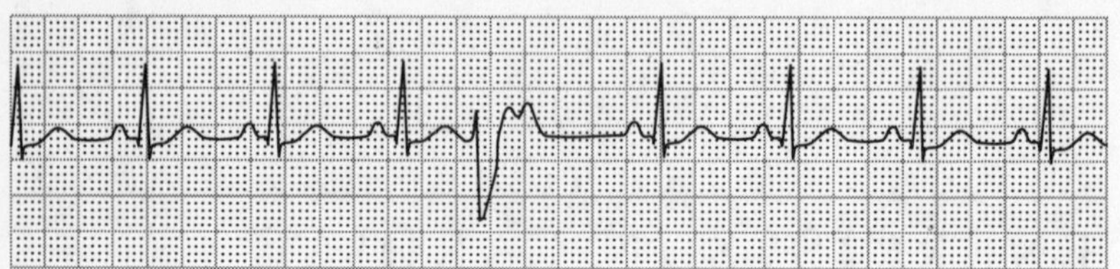

Rate Atrial:

Ventricular:

Rhythm Atrial:

Ventricular:

Conduction PR interval:

QRS complex:

Configuration and location P wave:

QRS complex:

T wave:

Rhythm interpretation:

Exercise 2

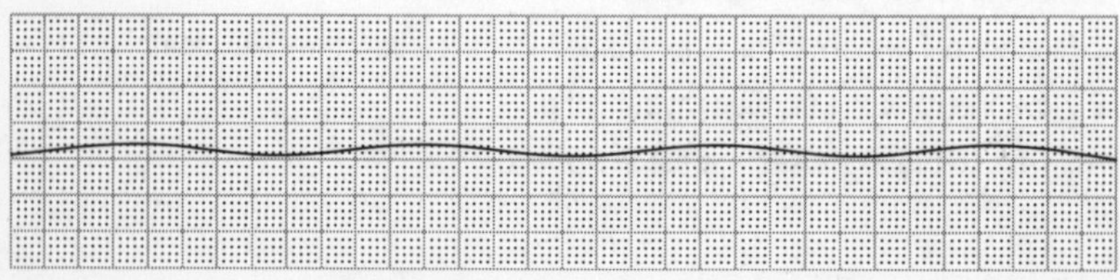

Rate Atrial:

Ventricular:

Rhythm Atrial:

Ventricular:

Conduction PR interval:

QRS complex:

Configuration and location P wave:

QRS complex:

T wave:

Rhythm interpretation:

Exercise 3

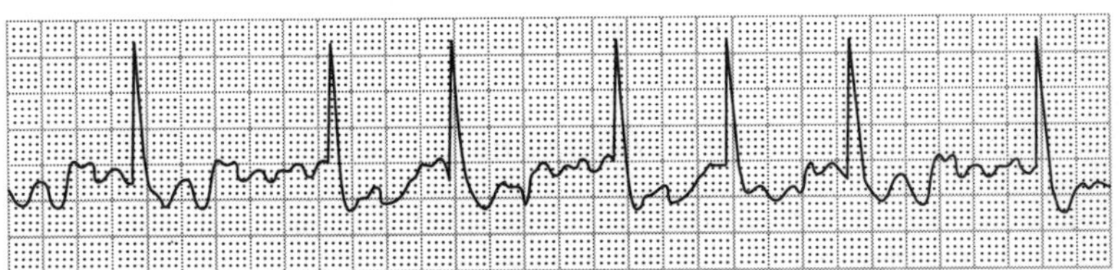

Rate Atrial:

Ventricular:

Rhythm Atrial:

Ventricular:

Conduction PR interval:

QRS complex:

Configuration and location P wave:

QRS complex:

T wave:

Rhythm interpretation:

Exercise 4

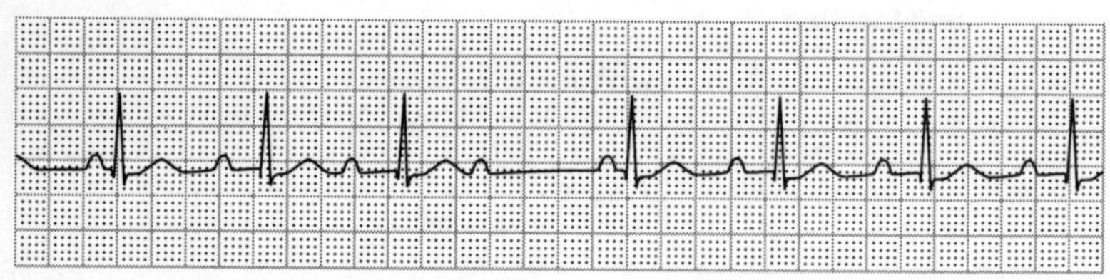

Rate Atrial:

Ventricular:

Rhythm Atrial:

Ventricular:

Conduction PR interval:

QRS complex:

Configuration and location P wave:

QRS complex:

T wave:

Rhythm interpretation:

Exercise 5

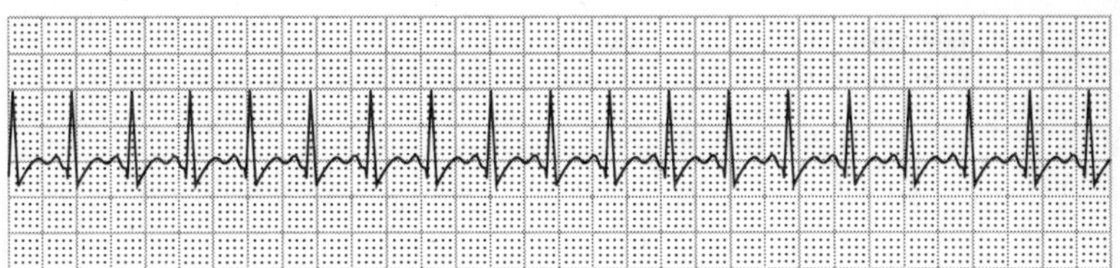

Rate	Atrial:
	Ventricular:
Rhythm	Atrial:
	Ventricular:
Conduction	PR interval:
	QRS complex:
Configuration and location	P wave:
	QRS complex:
	T wave:

Rhythm interpretation:

Exercise 6

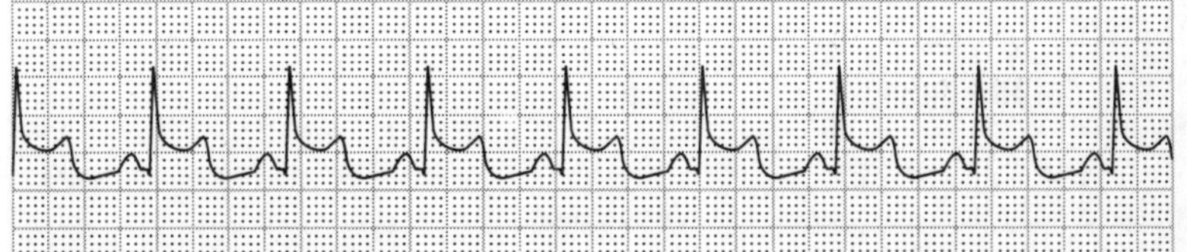

Rate Atrial:

Ventricular:

Rhythm Atrial:

Ventricular:

Conduction PR interval:

QRS complex:

Configuration and location P wave:

QRS complex:

T wave:

Rhythm interpretation:

Exercise 7

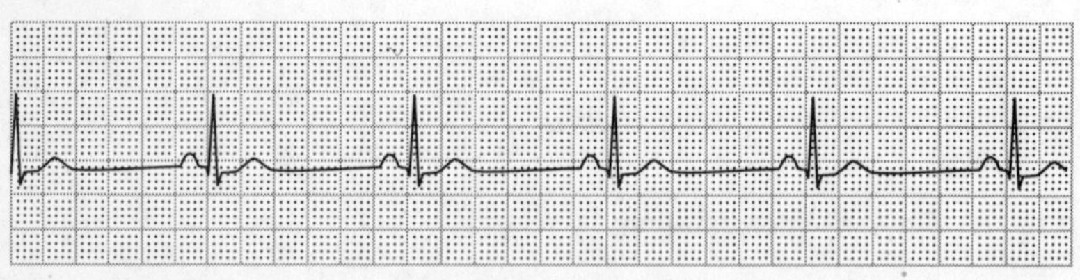

Rate Atrial:

Ventricular:

Rhythm Atrial:

Ventricular:

Conduction PR interval:

QRS complex:

Configuration and location P wave:

QRS complex:

T wave:

Rhythm interpretation:

Exercise 8

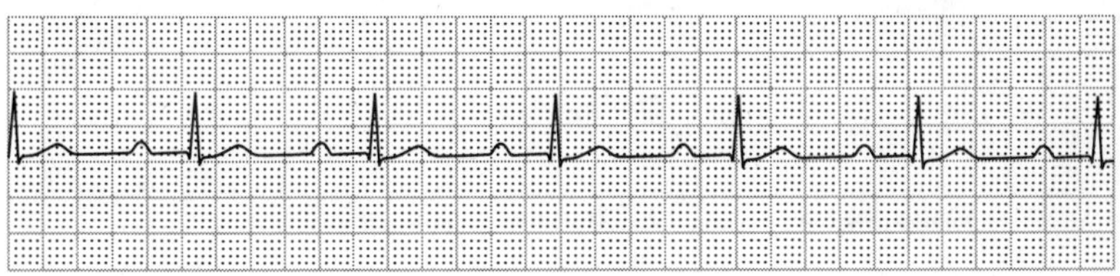

Rate Atrial:

Ventricular:

Rhythm Atrial:

Ventricular:

Conduction PR interval:

QRS complex:

Configuration and location P wave:

QRS complex:

T wave:

Rhythm interpretation:

Exercise 9

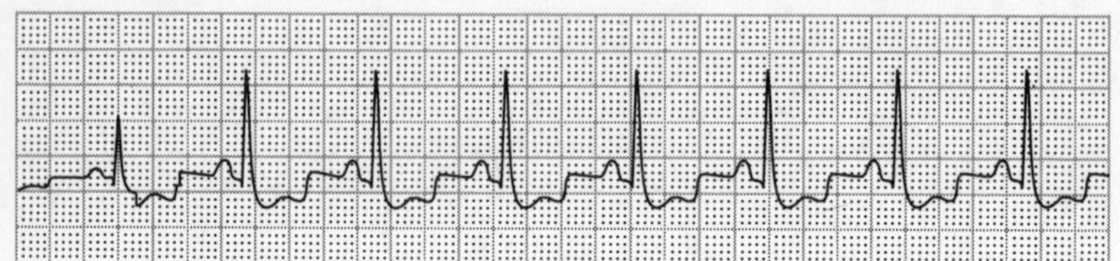

Rate Atrial:

Ventricular:

Rhythm Atrial:

Ventricular:

Conduction PR interval:

QRS complex:

Configuration and location P wave:

QRS complex:

T wave:

Rhythm interpretation:

Exercise 10

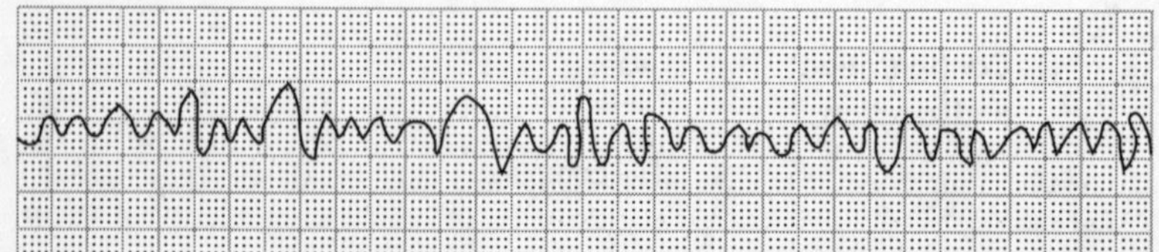

Rate	Atrial:
	Ventricular:
Rhythm	Atrial:
	Ventricular:
Conduction	PR interval:
	QRS complex:
Configuration and location	P wave:
	QRS complex:
	T wave:

Rhythm interpretation:

Exercise 11

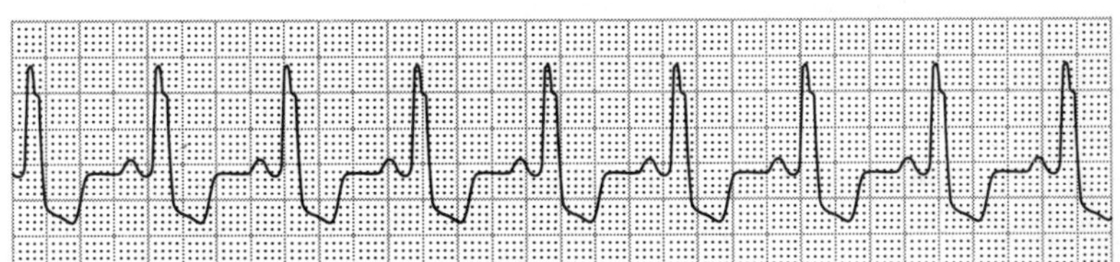

Rate	Atrial:
	Ventricular:
Rhythm	Atrial:
	Ventricular:
Conduction	PR interval:
	QRS complex:

Configuration and location P wave:

QRS complex:

T wave:

Rhythm interpretation:

Exercise 12

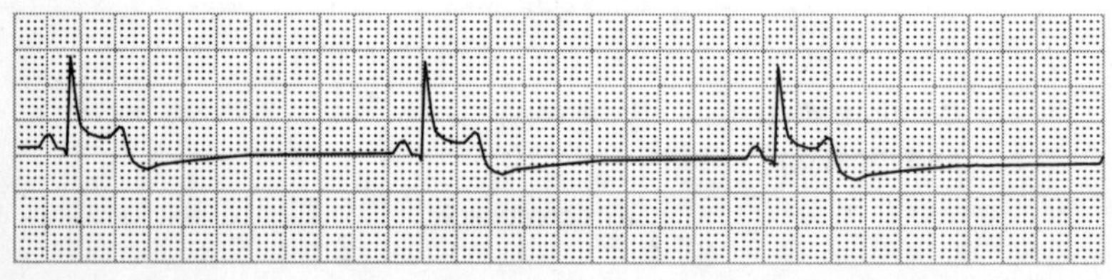

Rate Atrial:

Ventricular:

Rhythm Atrial:

Ventricular:

Conduction PR interval:

QRS complex:

Configuration and location P wave:

QRS complex:

T wave:

Rhythm interpretation:

Exercise 13

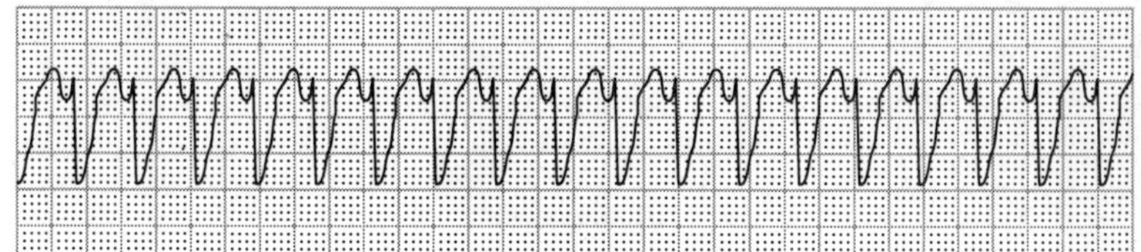

Rate Atrial:

Ventricular:

Rhythm Atrial:

Ventricular:

Conduction PR interval:

QRS complex:

Configuration and location P wave:

QRS complex:

T wave:

Rhythm interpretation:

Exercise 14

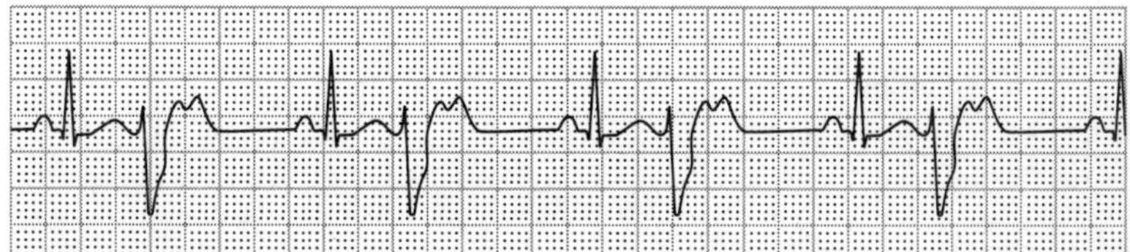

Rate Atrial:

Ventricular:

Rhythm Atrial:

Ventricular:

Conduction PR interval:

QRS complex:

Configuration and location P wave:

QRS complex:

T wave:

Rhythm interpretation:

Exercise 15

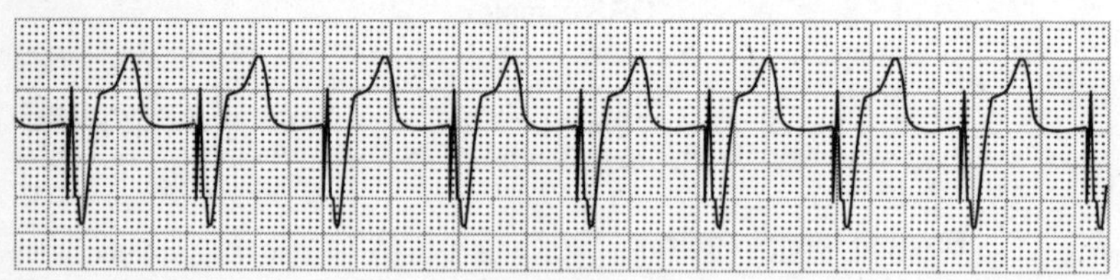

Rate Atrial:

Ventricular:

Rhythm Atrial:

Ventricular:

Conduction PR interval:

QRS complex:

Configuration and location P wave:

QRS complex:

T wave:

Rhythm interpretation:

Exercise 16

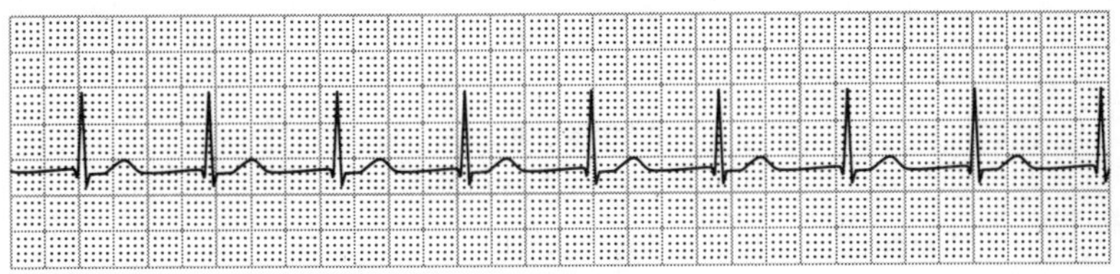

Rate Atrial:

Ventricular:

Rhythm Atrial:

Ventricular:

Conduction PR interval:

QRS complex:

Configuration and location P wave:

QRS complex:

T wave:

Rhythm interpretation:

Exercise 17

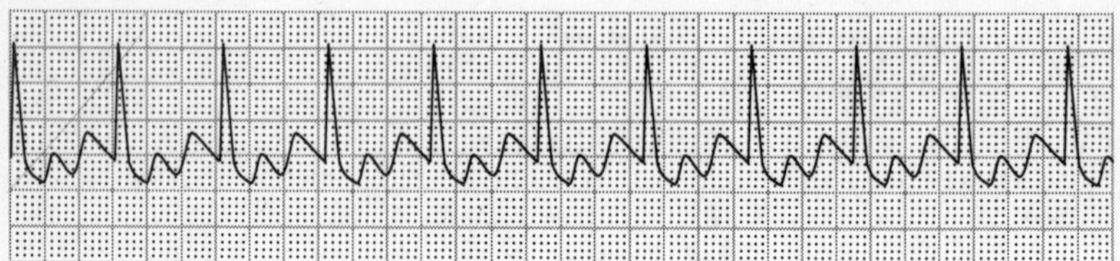

Rate Atrial:

Ventricular:

Rhythm Atrial:

Ventricular:

Conduction PR interval:

QRS complex:

Configuration and location P wave:

QRS complex:

T wave:

Rhythm interpretation:

Exercise 18

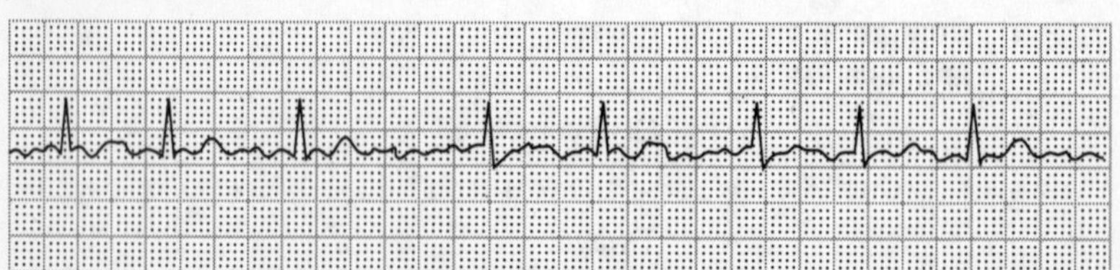

Rate	Atrial:
	Ventricular:
Rhythm	Atrial:
	Ventricular:
Conduction	PR interval:
	QRS complex:
Configuration and location	P wave:
	QRS complex:
	T wave:

Rhythm interpretation:

Exercise 19

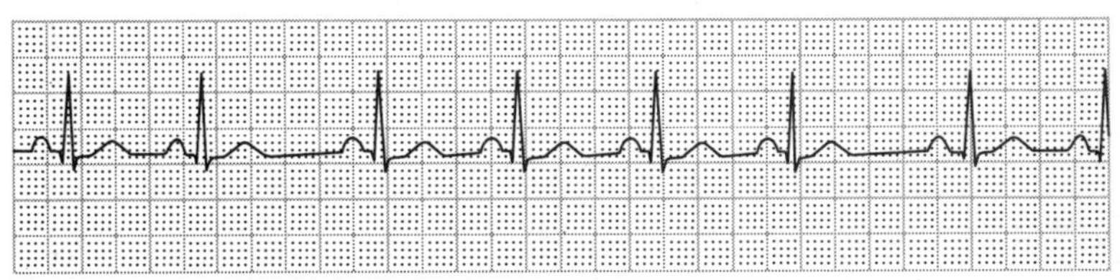

Rate	Atrial:
	Ventricular:
Rhythm	Atrial:
	Ventricular:

Conduction PR interval:

QRS complex:

Configuration and location P wave:

QRS complex:

T wave:

Rhythm interpretation:

Exercise 20

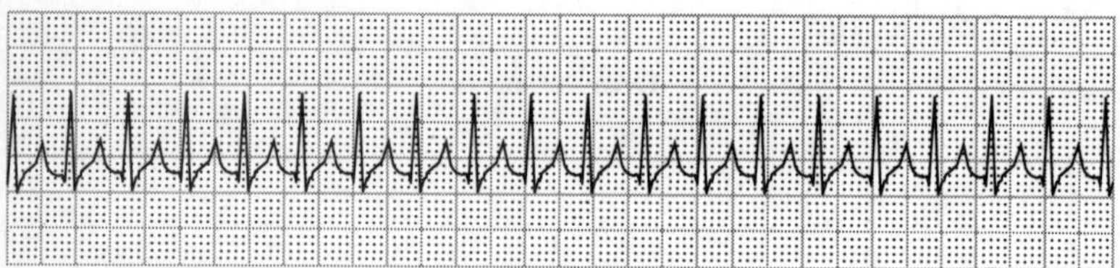

Rate Atrial:

Ventricular:

Rhythm Atrial:

Ventricular:

Conduction PR interval:

QRS complex:

Configuration and location P wave:

QRS complex:

T wave:

Rhythm interpretation:

Exercise 21

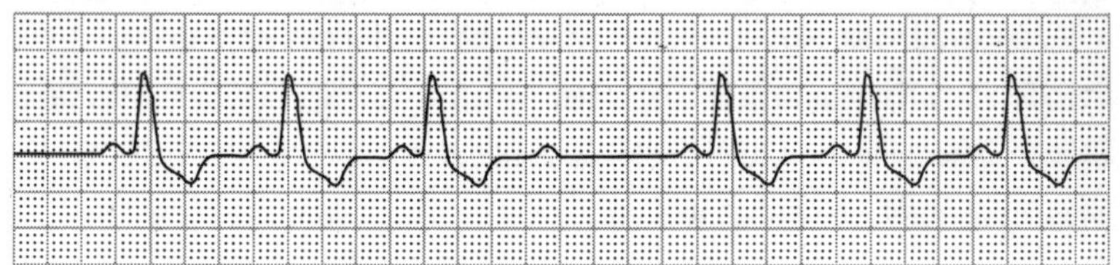

Rate Atrial:

Ventricular:

Rhythm Atrial:

Ventricular:

Conduction PR interval:

QRS complex:

Configuration and location P wave:

QRS complex:

T wave:

Rhythm interpretation:

PART B — 12 LEAD ECG INTERPRETATION

Step 1 Using the seven steps to interpret an MI as described in Chapter 6, analyse the following six 12 lead ECGs. Each of the traces were recorded when the patient was first admitted to the hospital. There are no consecutive traces for comparison on each of the patients and their clinical history is unknown.

Step 2 Ensure that all the leads have been recorded and that the trace is clear (all waves should be clearly visible). Has the ECG been standardised? Is there a recording of the patient's cardiac rhythm at the bottom of the page?

Step 3 Are there any ECG signs suggesting that the patient has had a myocardial infarction, that is, is there evidence of ST segment elevation greater than 1 mm or a presence of pathological Q waves?

Step 4 Look for reciprocal changes on the ECG (ST segment despression or a flat appearance). Note the leads where these changes appear.

Step 5 You will not be able to do this step because there is insufficient information.

Step 6 Determine the site of the MI (if any) and interpret the 12 lead ECG.

Step 7 Interpret the cardiac rhythm.

Answers to the exercises appear in Appendix 2.

Exercise 1

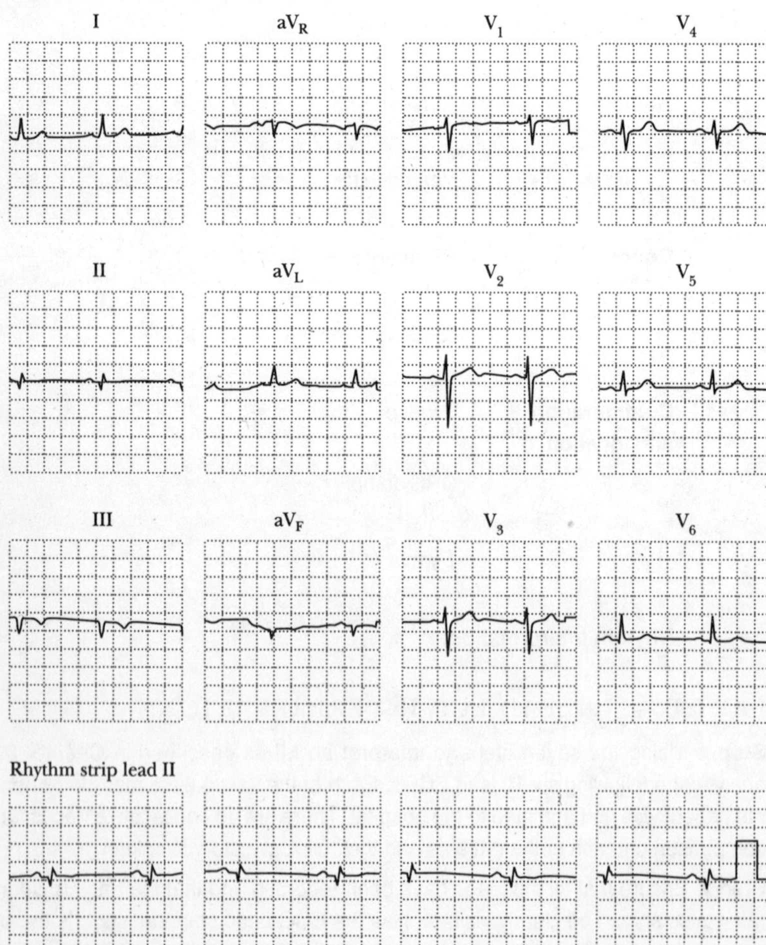

Exercise 2

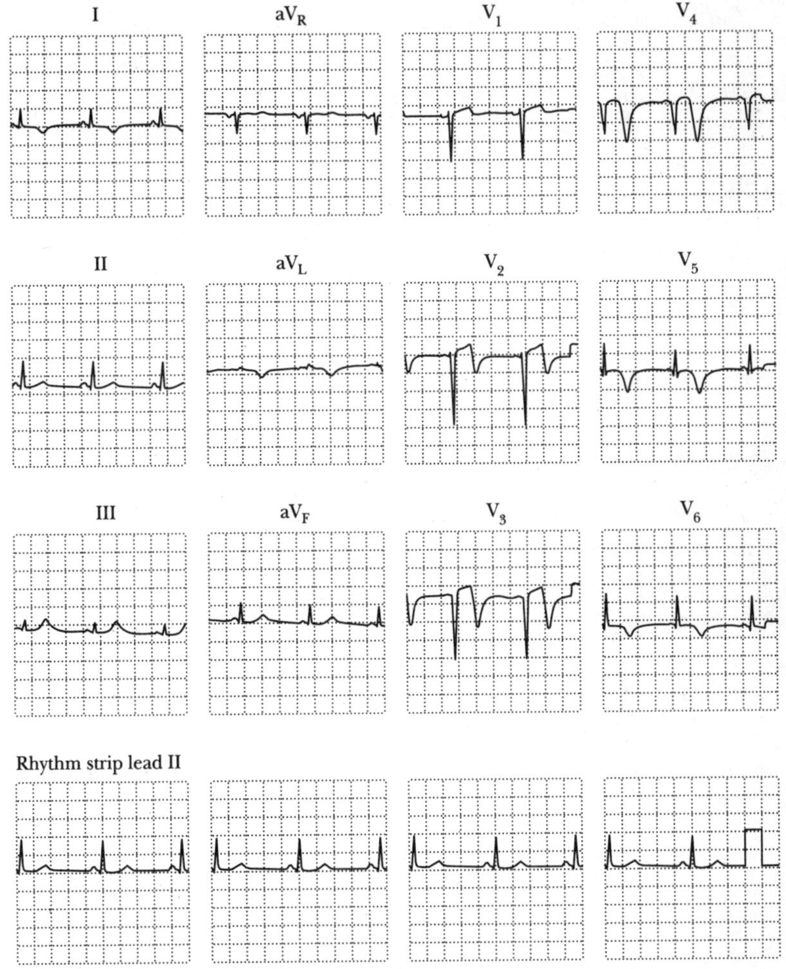
I
aVR
V1
V4
II
aVL
V2
V5
III
aVF
V3
V6
Rhythm strip lead II

Exercise 3

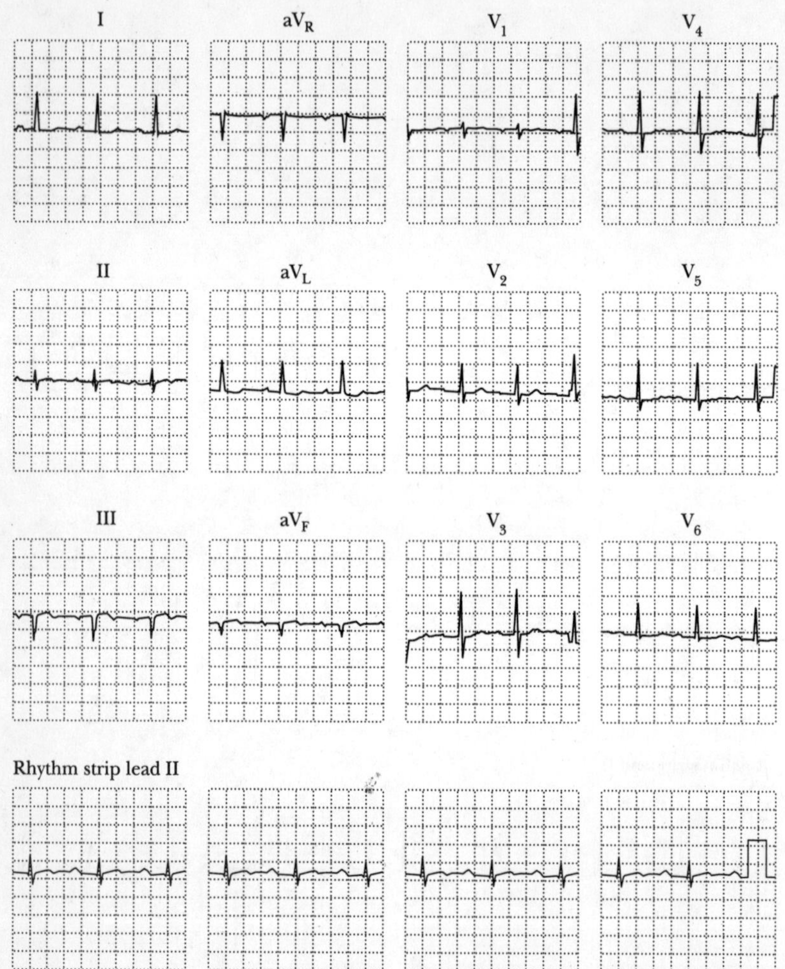
I
aVR
V1
V4
II
aVL
V2
V5
III
aVF
V3
V6
Rhythm strip lead II

Exercise 4

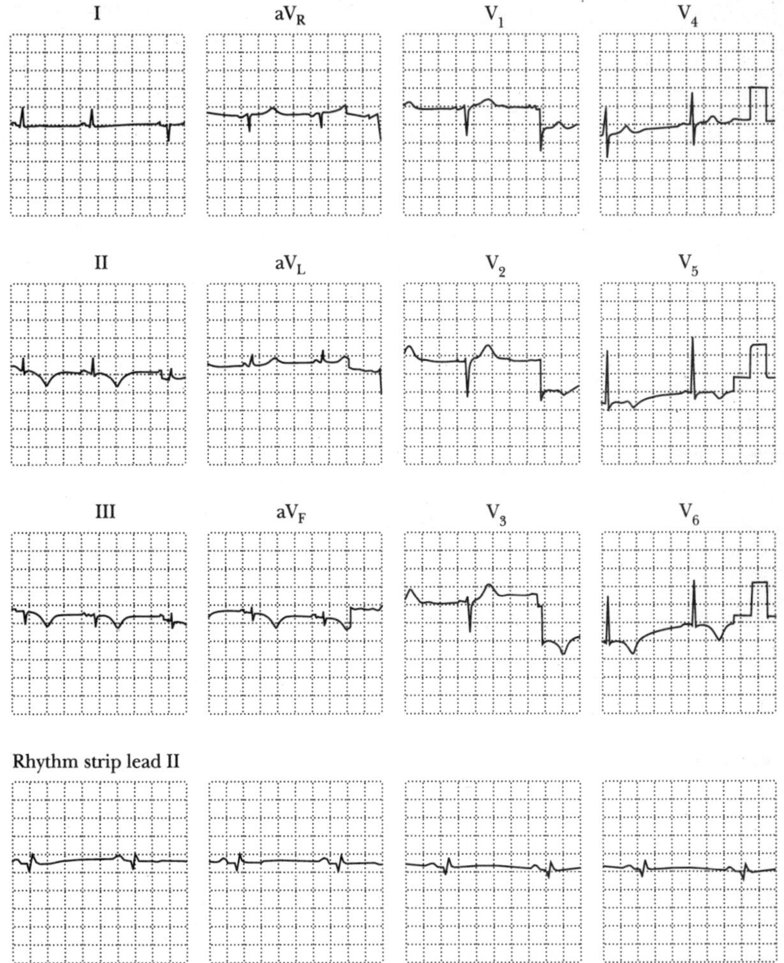
I
aV$_R$
V$_1$
V$_4$
II
aV$_L$
V$_2$
V$_5$
III
aV$_F$
V$_3$
V$_6$
Rhythm strip lead II

Exercise 5

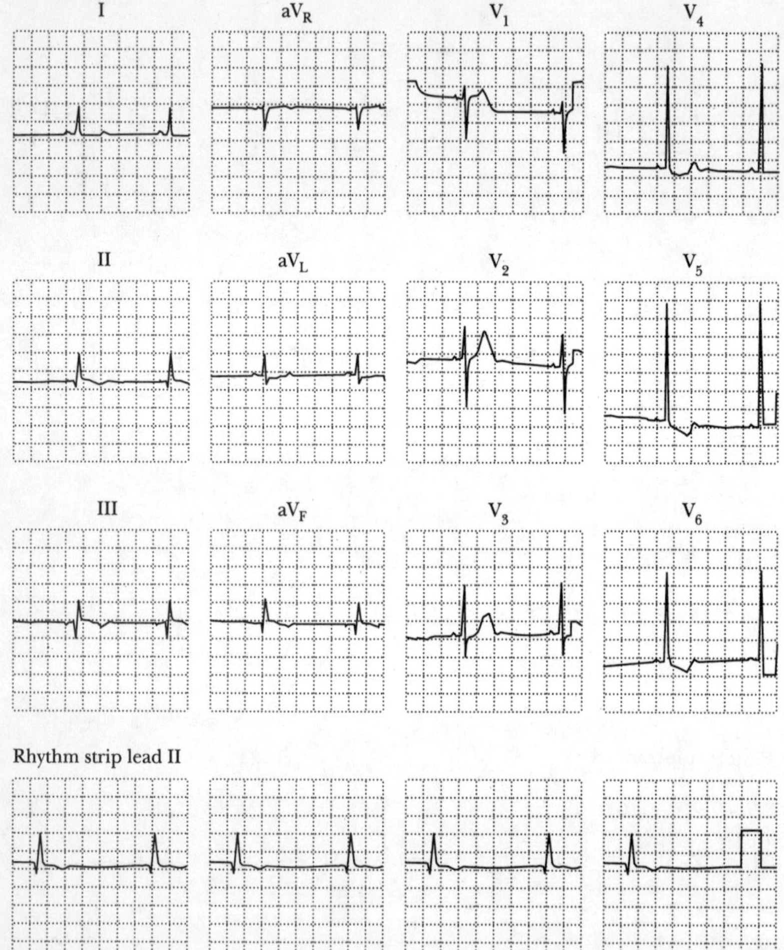
I
aV$_R$
V$_1$
V$_4$
II
aV$_L$
V$_2$
V$_5$
III
aV$_F$
V$_3$
V$_6$
Rhythm strip lead II

Exercise 6

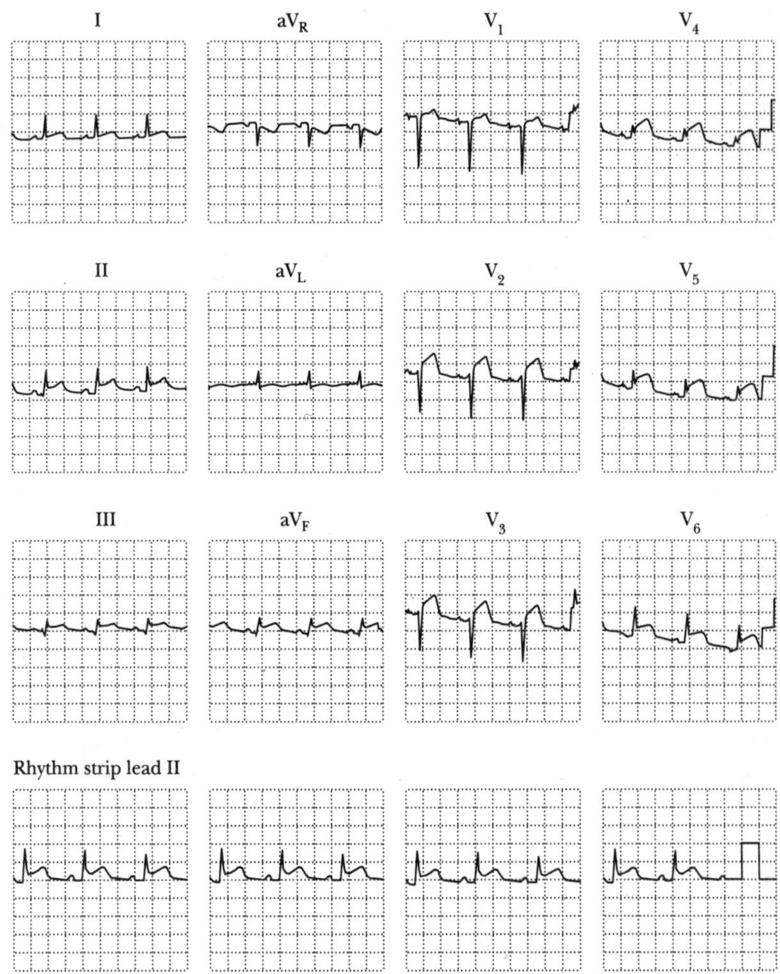
I
aVR
V1
V4
II
aVL
V2
V5
III
aVF
V3
V6
Rhythm strip lead II

APPENDIX 1

ANSWERS TO EXERCISES (CHAPTER 4)

Exercise 1

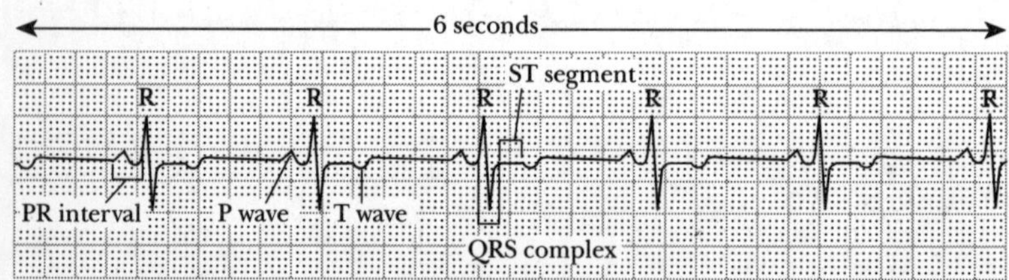

1 The **heart rate**:

 (i) In a six-second strip, the ventricular rate is approximately 50 bpm (RR cycles); or approximately 60 bpm (R waves only).

 (ii) Using the ECG ruler, the ventricular rate is approximately 55 bpm.

 (iii) Using the heavy dark lines, the heart rate is approximately 53 bpm.

 With heart rates of less than 60 bpm, the heavy dark line method is not as accurate as the other methods.

2 Looking at the **cardiac rhythm**, it appears to be regular. Use of the blank paper method to map the RR cycles confirms that it is regular.

3 The **P waves** are present and they all have a similar shape (upright, pointed and preceding the QRS complex).

4 The **PR interval** is approximately 0.16–0.18 seconds in duration and is within the normal range.

5 The **QRS complex** measures 0.12 seconds, even though the Q wave is not visible.

6 The **ST segment** is rounded and slightly depressed. A full 12 lead ECG would yield more information concerning the reasons for the shape of the ST segment. The patient may have had an MI, but this could only be interpreted from a 12 lead ECG.

7 The **T wave** is inverted and follows the QRS complex.

8 The **cardiac rhythm** is sinus bradycardia because the impulse originates in the SA node (presence of the P wave), and the PR interval and the QRS complex are within normal limits, indicating that the impulse has followed the normal conduction pathway within the required time frame. The heart rate is slow and regular.

Exercise 2

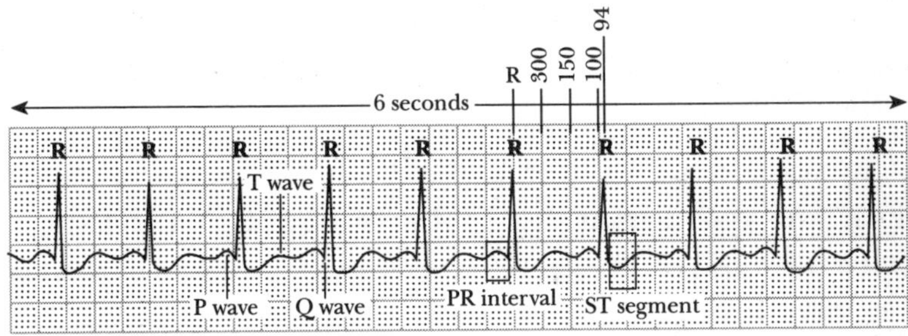

1 The **heart rate**:

(i) The ventricular heart rate is approximately 90 bpm using the six-second strip and the RR cycles. If just the R waves are counted, then the rate is 100 bpm.

(ii) Using the ECG ruler, the ventricular rate is approximately 95 bpm.

(iii) The heavy dark line approach yields an approximate heart rate of 94 bpm.

2 Using the blank piece of paper method to map the R waves, the **rhythm** is irregular and there are slight irregularities apparent at the fourth, sixth and eighth R waves.

3 The **P waves** are present, upright and rounded.

4 The **PR interval** is approximately 0.14 seconds in duration and within the normal range.

5 The **QRS complex** is approximately 0.06–0.08 seconds in duration and within the normal range.

6 The **ST segment** is depressed. A full 12 lead ECG would be helpful so that other leads could be visualised.

7 The **T wave** is present and follows the QRS complex and the ST segment.

8 The **cardiac rhythm** is normal sinus rhythm.

APPENDIX 2
ANSWERS TO EXERCISES
(CHAPTER 7)

PART A — CARDIAC RHYTHM INTERPRETATION

(Note: heart rates are calculated by using all the vertical lines in the heavy dark line method.)

Exercise 1

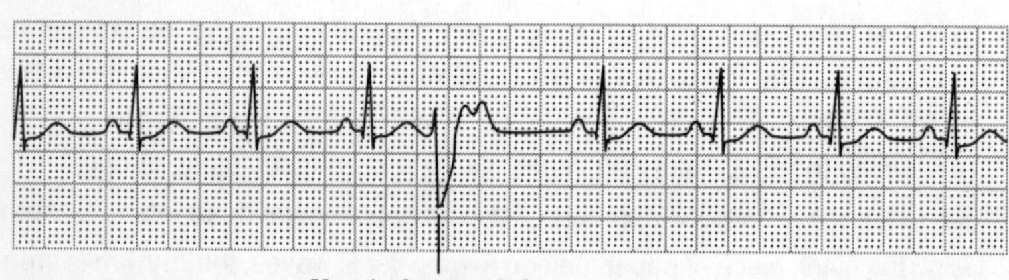

Ventricular ectopic beat

Rate	Atrial: 79 bpm Ventricular: 79 bpm
Rhythm	Atrial: regular (except for the ventricular ectopic beat) Ventricular: regular (except for the ventricular ectopic beat)
Conduction	PR interval: 0.18 seconds QRS complex: 0.06 seconds

Configuration and location	P wave: normal, before the QRS complex QRS complex: normal, after the P wave T wave: normal, after the QRS complex

Rhythm interpretation: sinus rhythm with one VEB

Exercise 2

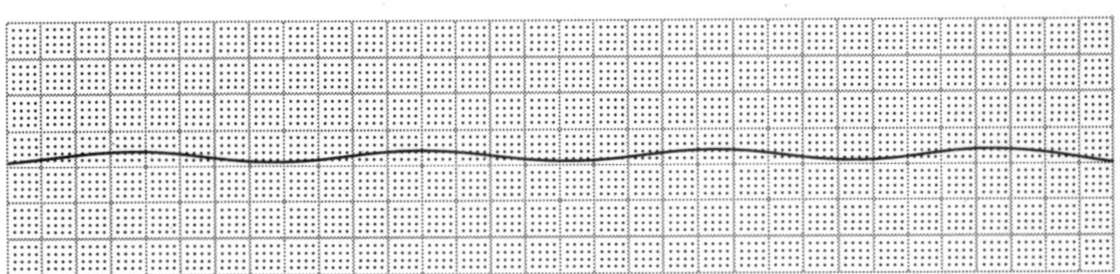

Rate	Atrial: not measurable Ventricular: not measurable
Rhythm	Atrial: not measurable Ventricular: not measurable
Conduction	PR interval: not measurable QT interval: not measurable
Configuration and location	P wave: none QRS complex: none T wave: none

Rhythm interpretation: ventricular standstill

Exercise 3

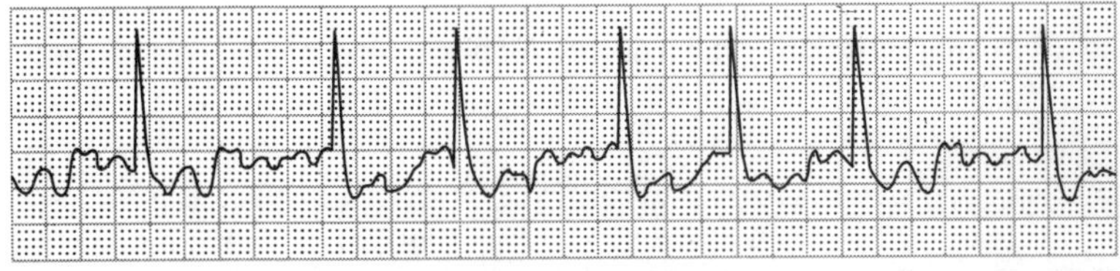

Rate	Atrial: too rapid to determine Ventricular: varies between 50 and 140 bpm
Rhythm	Atrial: irregular Ventricular: irregular

Conduction PR interval: not measurable
QRS complex: 0.06 seconds

Configuration and location P wave: chaotic, unidentifiable, no true P waves, f waves present
QRS complex: normal after the f waves
T wave: unidentifiable

Rhythm interpretation: atrial fibrillation

Exercise 4

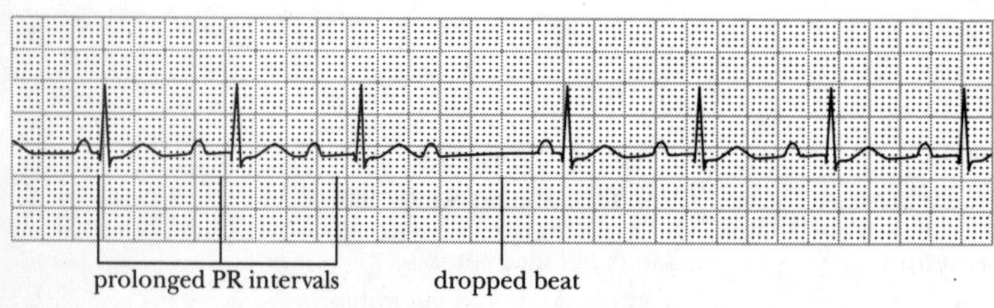

Rate Atrial: 80 bpm
Ventricular: 70 bpm

Rhythm Atrial: regular
Ventricular: irregular because of dropped QRS complex

Conduction PR interval: progressive lengthening
QRS complex: 0.06 seconds

Configuration and location P wave: normal, sometimes more than one
QRS complex: normal after the P waves, except for a dropped beat
T wave: normal

Rhythm interpretation: second degree AV block, Mobitz type I (Wenckebach)

Exercise 5

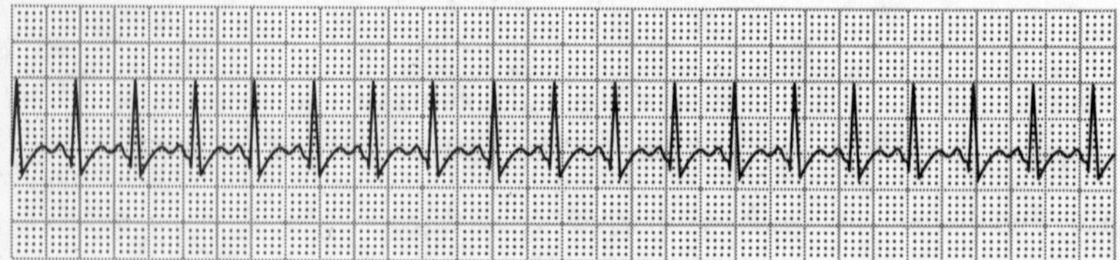

Rate	Atrial: 167 bpm Ventricular: 167 bpm
Rhythm	Atrial: regular Ventricular: regular
Conduction	PR interval: 0.12 seconds QRS complex: 0.08 seconds
Configuration and location	P wave: upright, rounded; precedes QRS complex QRS complex: normal T wave: normal and follows QRS complex; because of the fast rate the T wave has merged into the end of the ST segment
Rhythm interpretation:	sinus tachycardia

Exercise 6

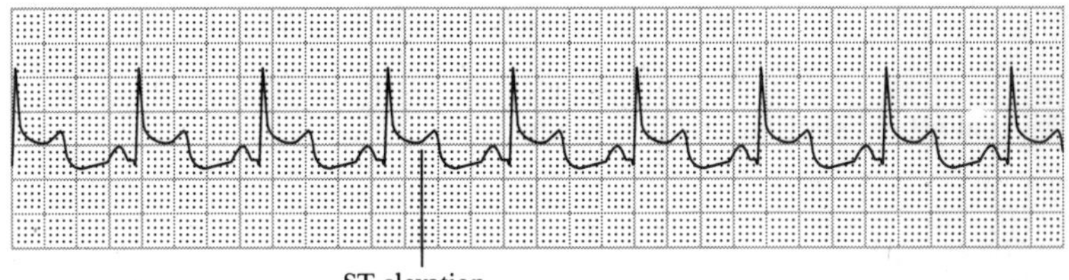

ST elevation

Rate	Atrial: 75 bpm Ventricular: 75 bpm
Rhythm	Atrial: regular Ventricular: regular
Conduction	PR interval: 0.16 seconds QRS complex: 0.06 seconds
Configuration and location	P wave: normal (upright, rounded) QRS complex: normal, but ST segment elevated T wave: caught up in the end of the ST segment
Rhythm interpretation:	sinus rhythm (ST elevation indicated by arrow); a 12 lead ECG would provide more information

Exercise 7

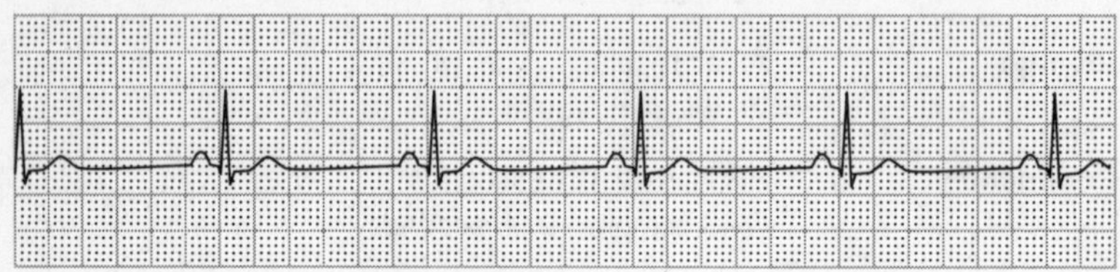

Rate	Atrial: 50 bpm Ventricular: 50 bpm
Rhythm	Atrial: regular Ventricular: regular
Conduction	PR interval: 0.16 seconds QRS complex: 0.06 seconds
Configuration and location	P wave: normal; precedes QRS complex QRS complex: narrow, but normal; follows p wave T wave: normal; follows ST segment

Rhythm interpretation: sinus bradycardia

Exercise 8

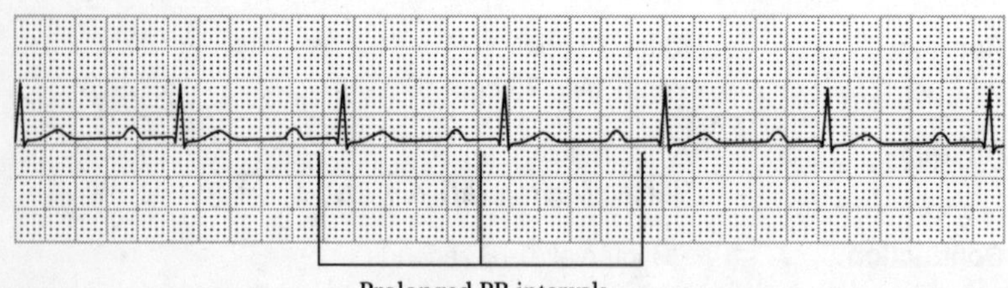

Rate	Atrial: 60 bpm Ventricular: 60 bpm
Rhythm	Atrial: regular Ventricular: regular
Conduction	PR interval: 0.34 seconds QRS complex: 0.06 seconds
Configuration and location	P wave: normal, before the QRS complex QRS complex: normal T wave: normal

Rhythm interpretation: sinus bradycardia with first degree AV block

Exercise 9

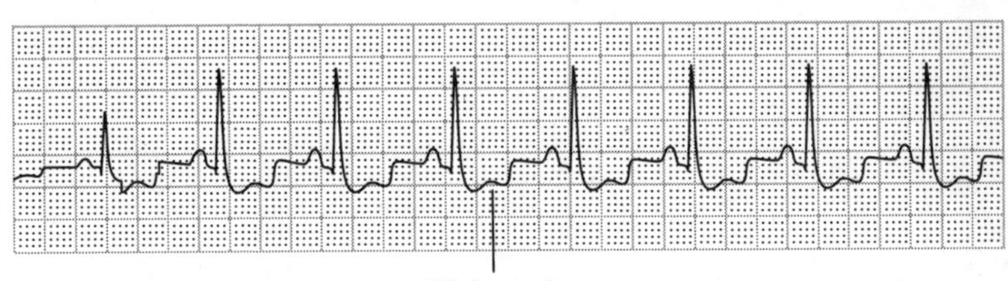

Rate	Atrial: 79 bpm Ventricular: 79 bpm
Rhythm	Atrial: regular Ventricular: regular
Conduction	PR interval: 0.18 seconds QRS complex: 0.08 seconds
Configuration and location	P wave: normal (upright, rounded) QRS complex: normal (upright) T wave: merges into the end of the depressed ST segment
Rhythm interpretation:	sinus rhythm (note the depressed ST segment). There is an ectopic beat at the beginning of the trace

Exercise 10

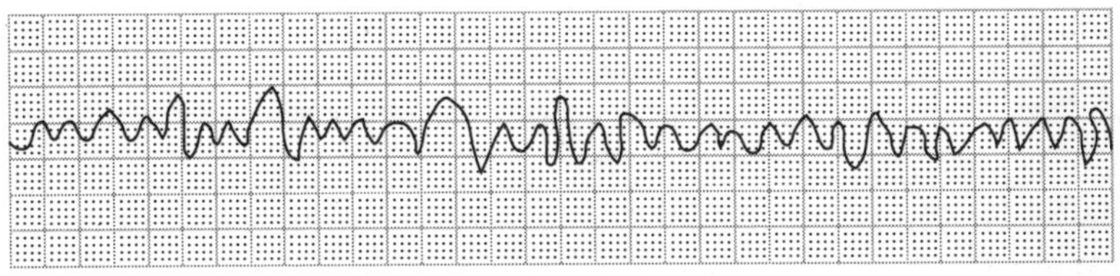

Rate	Atrial: no P waves Ventricular: no QRS complexes
Rhythm	Atrial: chaotic Ventricular: chaotic
Conduction	PR interval: absent QRS complex: absent

Configuration and location	P wave: absent QRS complex: absent T wave: absent
Rhythm interpretation:	ventricular fibrillation

Exercise 11

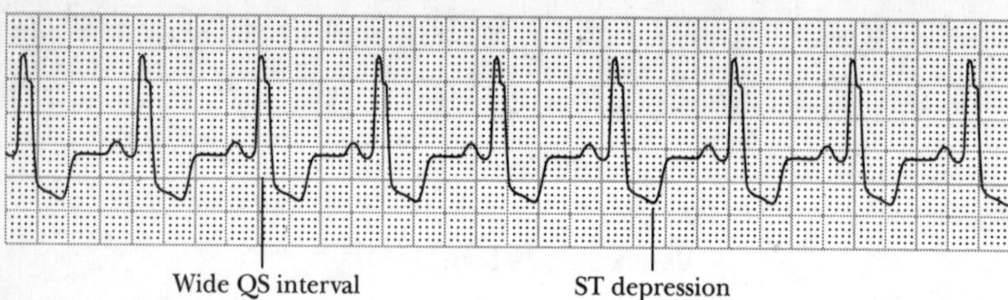

Rate	Atrial: 80 bpm Ventricular: 80 bpm
Rhythm	Atrial: regular Ventricular: regular
Conduction	PR interval: 0.16 seconds QRS complex: greater than 0.12 seconds
Configuration and location	P wave: normal (upright, rounded) QRS complex: depressed ST segment and wider QRS complex T wave: difficult to determine because of wider QRS complex
Rhythm interpretation:	sinus rhythm. Note the notching at the top of the R wave. There may be a bundle branch block present, but you would need to see the 12 lead ECG to determine whether it involves the left bundle branch or the right bundle branch

Exercise 12

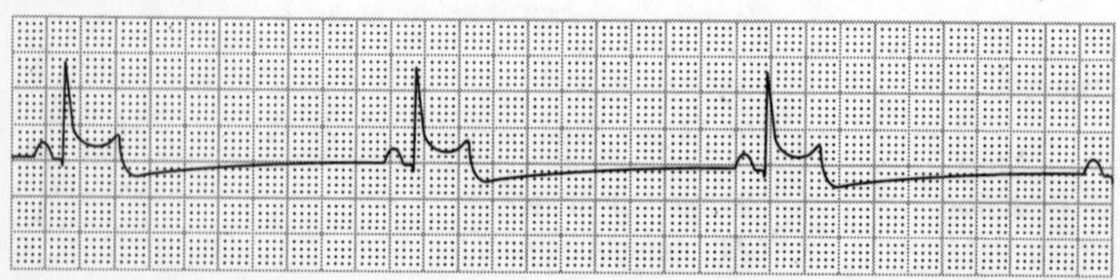

Rate	Atrial: 30 bpm Ventricular: 30 bpm
Rhythm	Atrial: regular Ventricular: regular
Conduction	PR interval: 0.16 seconds QRS complex: 0.08 seconds
Configuration and location	P wave: normal (upright), precedes QRS complex QRS complex: normal, except the ST segment is elevated T wave: merges with the end of the ST segment

Rhythm interpretation: sinus bradycardia. People with these rates may be symptomatic and may also need pacing

Exercise 13

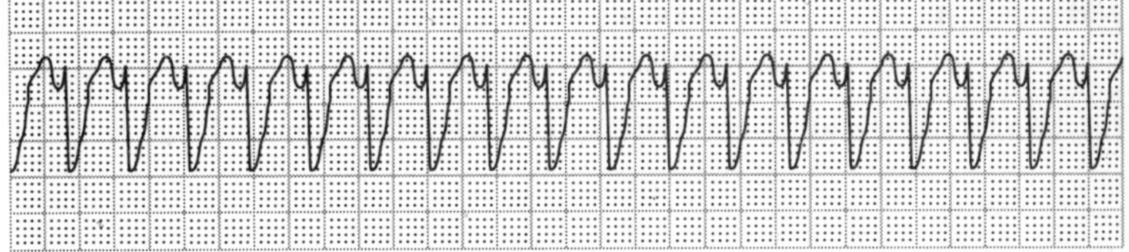

Rate	Atrial: not measurable; no P waves Ventricular: 187 bpm
Rhythm	Atrial: regular Ventricular: regular
Conduction	PR interval: absent QRS complex: greater than 0.12 seconds
Configuration and location	P wave: absent QRS complex: widened complex T wave: absent

Rhythm interpretation: ventricular tachycardia

Exercise 14

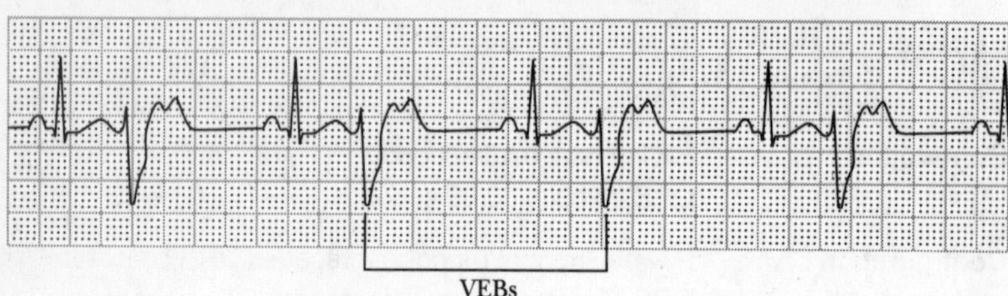

Rate	Atrial: 50 bpm Ventricular: 115 bpm
Rhythm	Atrial: no P waves before ventricular ectopic beats Ventricular: regular, except for ventricular ectopic beats
Conduction	PR interval: when present, 0.16 seconds QRS complex: 0.06 seconds in normal beats
Configuration and location	P wave: normal (upright, rounded) QRS complex: normal in normal complexes T wave: upright, rounded
Rhythm interpretation:	bigeminy; one normal PQRST followed by a ventricular ectopic beat

Exercise 15

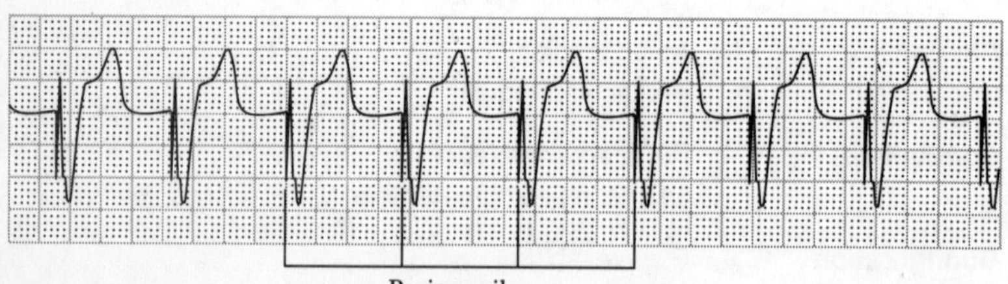

Rate	Atrial: paced rhythm Ventricular: 79 bpm
Rhythm	Atrial: paced rhythm Ventricular: paced rhythm
Conduction	PR interval: absent QRS complex: uniform interval

Configuration and location	P wave: not present QRS complex: wide, uniform; normal for paced rhythm T wave: not present
Rhythm interpretation:	paced rhythm. The patient has a temporary or permanent pacemaker insitu. (Note the pacing spikes)

Exercise 16

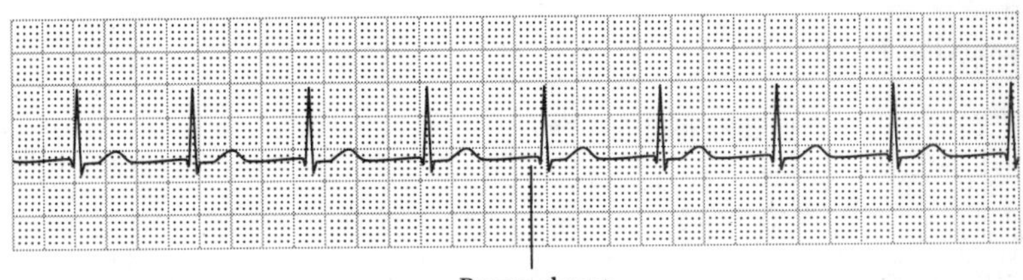

Rate	Atrial: P waves absent Ventricular: 79 bpm
Rhythm	Atrial: P waves absent Ventricular: regular
Conduction	PR interval: not measurable QRS complex: 0.06 seconds
Configuration and location	P wave: absent QRS complex: normal T wave: normal (upright, rounded)
Rhythm interpretation:	accelerated junctional rhythm

Exercise 17

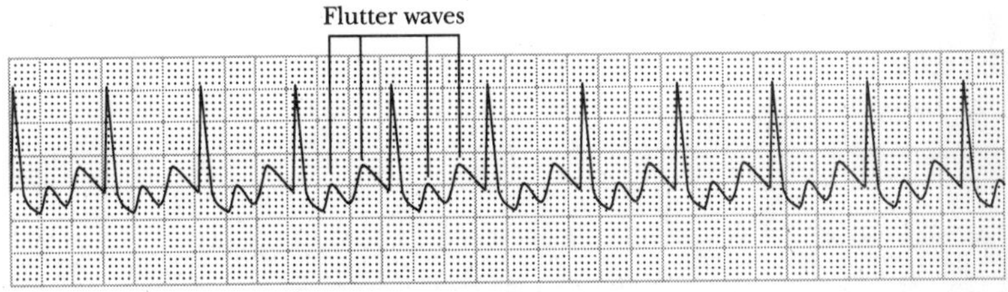

Rate	Atrial: 180–200 bpm Ventricular: 100 bpm
Rhythm	Atrial: regular Ventricular: regular

Conduction PR interval: absent
QRS complex: 0.08 seconds

Configuration and location P wave: no true P waves, only F waves
QRS complex: normal
T wave: absent

Rhythm interpretation: atrial flutter with 2:1 block

Exercise 18

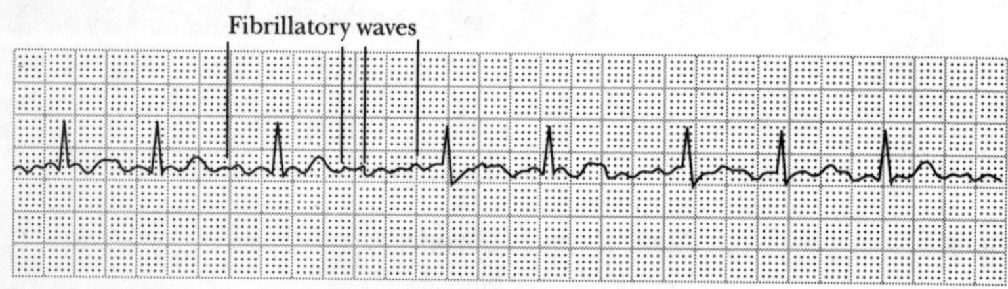

Rate Atrial: 300 bpm
Ventricular: 100 bpm

Rhythm Atrial: irregular, chaotic
Ventricular: irregular

Conduction PR interval: absent
QRS complex: 0.08 seconds

Configuration and location P wave: no true P waves, only f waves
QRS complex: normal
T wave: absent

Rhythm interpretation: atrial fibrillation

Exercise 19

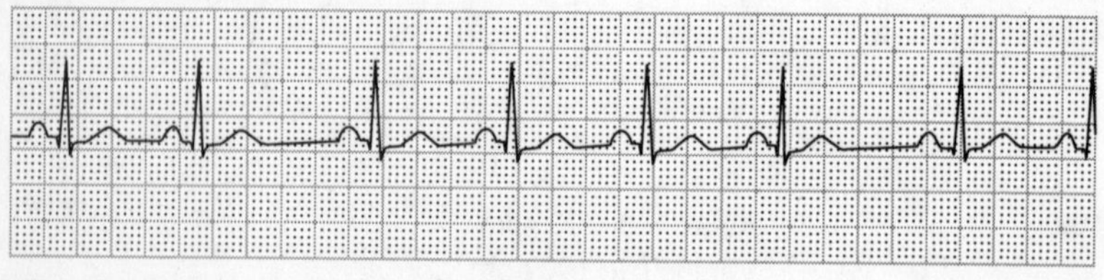

Rate Atrial: 60–80 bpm
Ventricular: 60–80 bpm

Rhythm	Atrial: irregular Ventricular: irregular
Conduction	PR interval: 0.14 seconds QRS complex: 0.06 seconds
Configuration and location	P wave: normal QRS complex: normal T wave: normal (upright, rounded)
Rhythm interpretation:	sinus arrhythmia (notice the effects of breathing)

Exercise 20

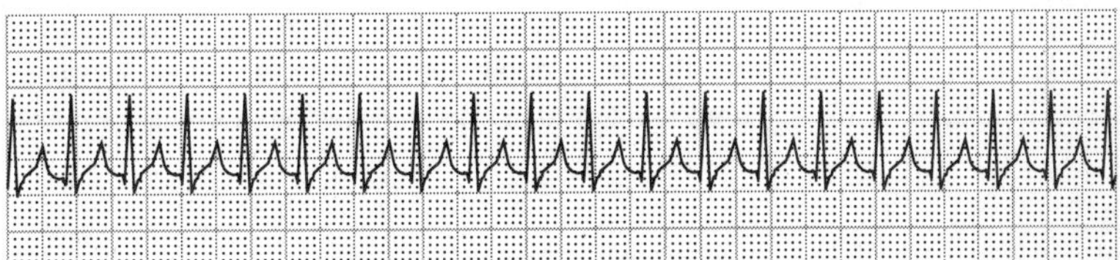

Rate	Atrial: cannot be determined as there are no P waves Ventricular: 187 bpm
Rhythm	Atrial: cannot be determined Ventricular: regular
Conduction	PR interval: none QRS complex: 0.08 seconds
Configuration and location	P wave: absent QRS complex: normal T wave: pointed and upright because of fast rate
Rhythm interpretation:	paroxysmal atrial tachycardia or paroxysmal junctional tachycardia

Exercise 21

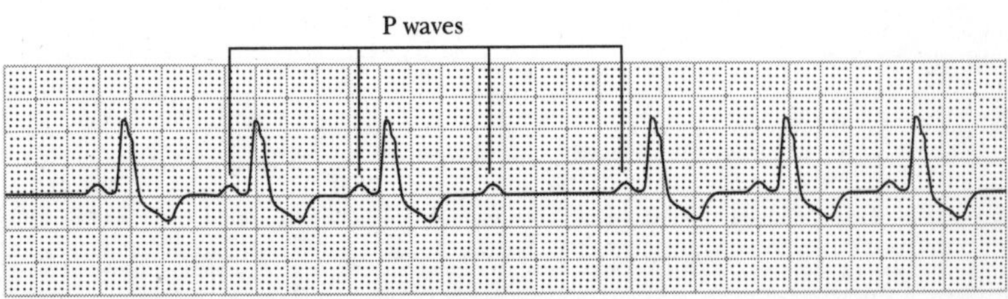

Rate	Atrial: 75 bpm, except for dropped beat Ventricular: 75 bpm, except for dropped beat
Rhythm	Atrial: regular PP intervals Ventricular: irregular because of the dropped beat
Conduction	PR interval: 0.20 seconds QRS complex: greater than 0.12 seconds
Configuration and location	P wave: normal (upright, rounded) QRS complex: widened; notching at top of R wave T wave: merges with slurred ST segment
Rhythm interpretation:	there is a wider QRS complex (greater than 0.12 seconds) and a dropped beat (QRS). There also appears to have been a dropped beat before the QRS complex. The rhythm is Mobitz type II second degree AV block. There is a 2:1 block present (two P waves to one QRS complex)

PART B — 12 LEAD ECG INTERPRETATION

Exercise 1

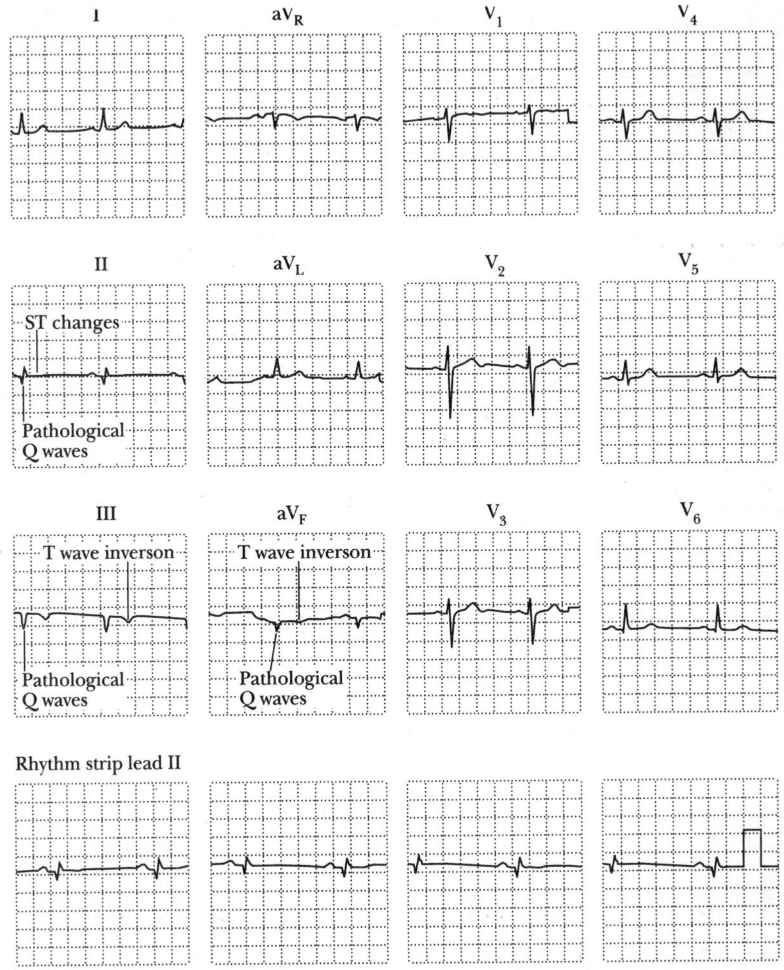

There are pathological Q waves in LII, LIII, and aV$_F$, as well as some ST segment changes. LII and aV$_F$ are flat and in LIII the T wave is inverted. There is evidence of inverted T waves developing in the anterior leads. The patient has had an inferior MI with reciprocal changes in the anterior leads. The cardiac rhythm is sinus bradycardia.

Exercise 2

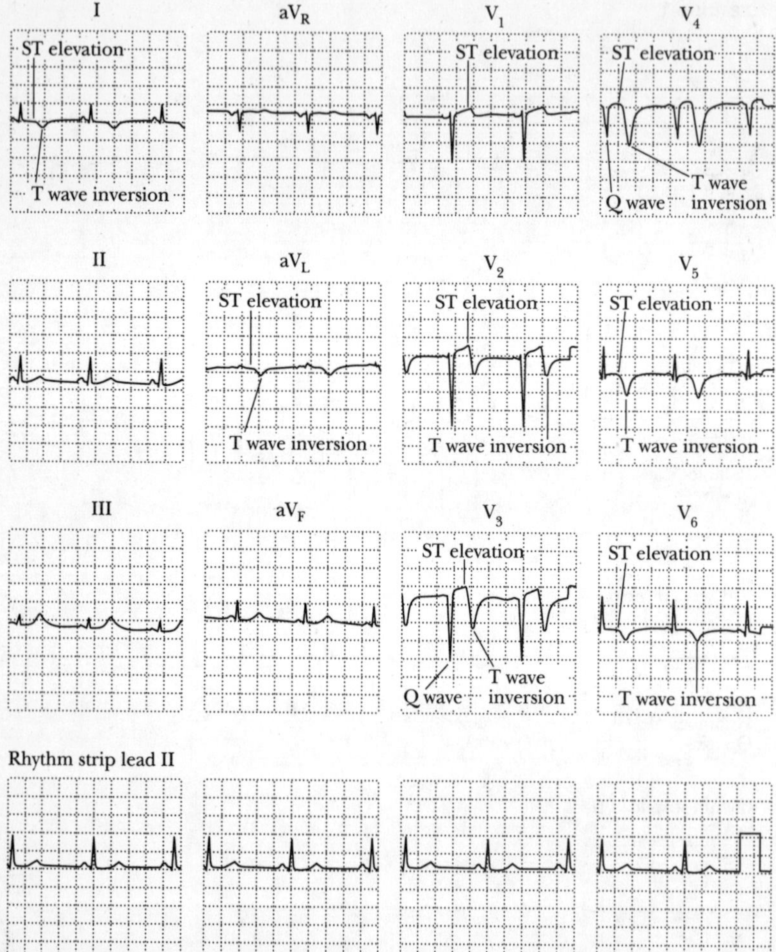

There is ST segment elevation in leads V_1–V_6, LI and aV_L. Deep symmetrical T wave inversion exists in V_1–V_6, LI and aV_L. There is slight ST segment depression in the inferior leads (LII, LIII and aV_F). There are Q waves in V_3 and V_4. The patient has probably had an anterior/ lateral MI approximately two days ago. The cardiac rhythm is normal sinus rhythm.

Exercise 3

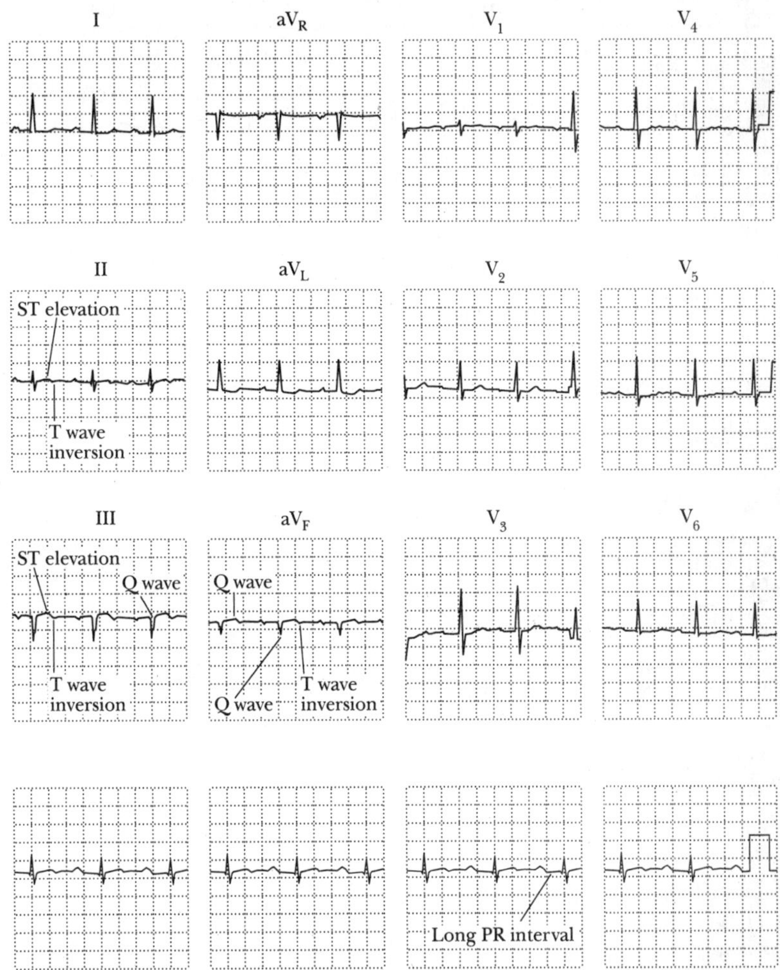

There is slight ST elevation in the inferior leads, LII, LIII and aV$_F$, and ischaemic changes in the anterior lateral leads. This is characterised by ST segment depression and a slightly inverted T wave. The patient has probably had an inferior MI. The cardiac rhythm is sinus rhythm with first degree AV block — note that the prolonged PR interval equals 0.30 seconds.

Exercise 4

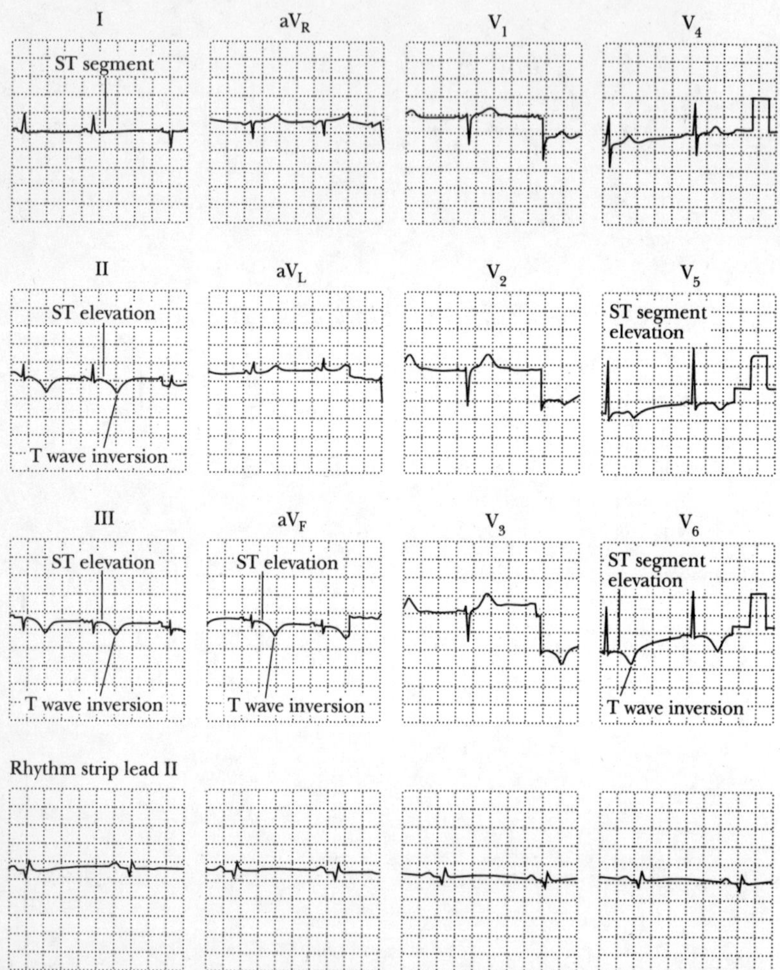

There is deep symmetrical T wave inversion in the inferior lateral leads (LI, LII, LIII, aV$_F$, V$_5$ and V$_6$). The initial impression is that the patient has an inferior/lateral myocardial ischaemia, though it is quite probable that this patient did have an inferior/lateral MI. There is no cardiac rhythm strip recorded, but the patient is in sinus bradycardia.

Exercise 5

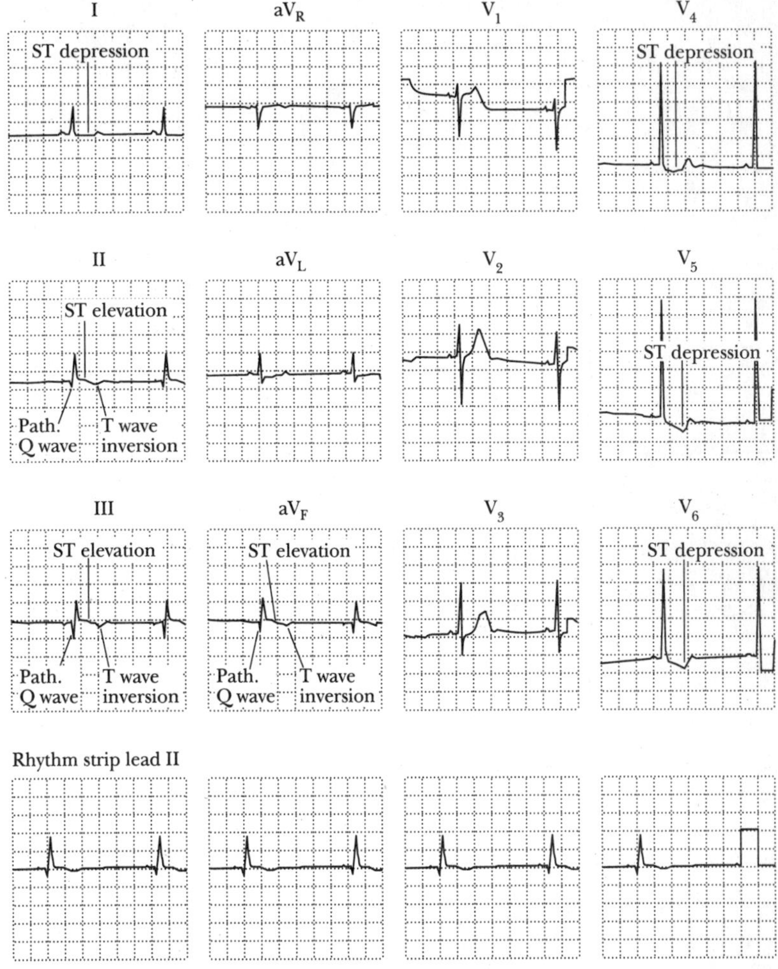

There are pathological Q waves in the inferior leads, LII, LIII and aV_F, and there is ST elevation as well as T wave inversion in the inferior leads. In the lateral leads there is ST segment depression (LI, aV_L, V_5, V_6, as well as V_4). The patient has had an inferior MI with reciprocal changes in the lateral leads. The cardiac rhythm is sinus bradycardia. Note the tall QRS complexes in V_4, V_5 and V_6. Add the depth of the S wave (in mm) in V_1 to the height of the R wave (in mm) in V_5 (which equals 54 mm). If the result is more than 35 mm, this is indicative of left ventricular hyperthrophy.

Exercise 6

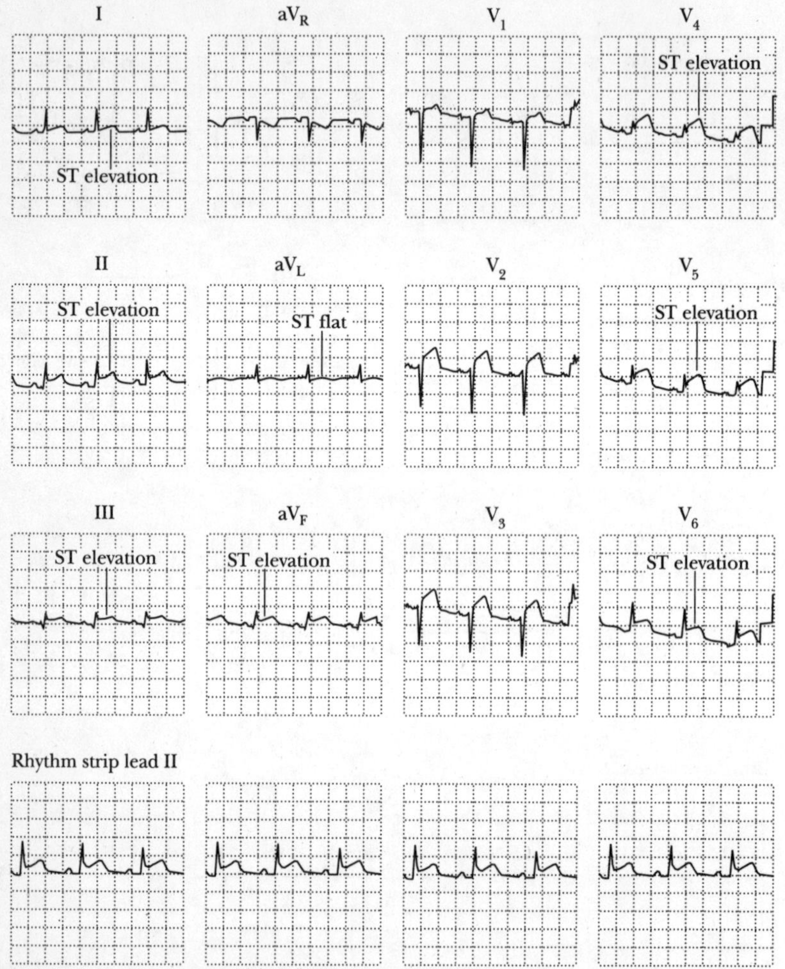

There is ST elevation in LII, LIII, aV$_F$, V$_2$–V$_6$ and LI. The ST segment in aV$_L$ is flat. The patient has probably had an inferior/lateral MI. The cardiac rhythm is sinus rhythm.

GLOSSARY

12 lead electrocardiogram (ECG)
A graph of the electrical activity of the heart. A 12 lead ECG is obtained by placing electrodes on specific sites of the patient's body. In turn, these are connected to a machine via leads. It is a non-invasive procedure.

Absolute refractory period
When the heart is in a state of contraction.

Action potential
The cell's ability to respond to an electrical stimulus. At a physiological level, it is the movement of ions across a semipermeable membrane resulting in the phases of depolarisation and repolarisation of the myocardial cell.

Advanced life support (ALS)
Stabilisation of cardiopulmonary functions by airway intubation and oxygenation, administration of intravenous fluid and medications, and initiating defibrillation.

Afterload
The amount of resistance which the ventricles have to work against to effectively eject blood into the pulmonary or systemic circulation.

Ambulatory monitoring
A means of recording the patient's cardiac rhythm while they are performing their daily activities. Ambulatory monitoring is used for the detection of abnormal rhythm patterns and to evaluate the effectiveness of medication.

Aneurysm
A dilatation in the wall of an artery, vein or a chamber of the heart.

Antiarrhythmic medications
Pharmacological agents used in the treatment of arrhythmias.

Aortic valve
Separates the left ventricle from the aorta.

Arrhythmia
An alteration or an irregularity in the pulse rhythm. Some texts use the term *dysrhythmia*.

Arteriole
A terminal artery that feeds directly into a capillary.

Aspartate transaminase
A cardiac enzyme which becomes elevated following a myocardial infarction. Aspartate transaminase is measured to confirm the diagnosis.

Asynchronised
The delivery of an electrical countershock without a QRS complex sensing device.

Atherosclerosis
A form of arteriosclerosis in which deposits of yellow plaque containing cholesterols and lipids are formed within the lining of large- and medium-sized arteries.

Atrioventricular (AV) node
Part of the heart's conduction system involved in the transmission of electrical impulses from the sinoatrial (SA) node. If the SA node should fail to emit an impulse at the required time, the AV node, or the tissue surrounding it, is capable of emitting an impulse at the rate of 60 bpm.

Atrioventricular universal pacing
A pacing mode associated with cardiac pacemakers. In this arrangement there is a pacing and sensing electrode in both chambers of the heart (atrium and ventricle).

Atrium
Upper chamber of the heart. There is an atrium on each side of the septum. The right atrium deals with deoxygenated blood returning from the body; the left atrium carries oxygenated blood. Both atriums act as reservoirs.

Auscultation
The practice of examining the body by listening to body sounds using a stethoscope.

Automaticity
The ability of cardiac muscle cells to reach a threshold potential and be able to generate an action potential without the need for external stimulation.

Bainbridge reflex
A nervous reflex which is activated when the right atrial walls are stretched. A Bainbridge reflex results in an increase in the heart rate.

Basic life support (BLS)
Constitutes an emergency airway, breathing, oxygenation and circulatory support following the ventilation–compression ratio.

Bifocal pacing
The pacemaker mode can pace both the atria and the ventricles when needed.

Bigeminy
A normal sinus beat followed by a ventricular ectopic beat.

Bipolar catheter
A type of pacing catheter which consists of a negative pacing electrode situated in the tip of the catheter, and a positive sensing electrode located approximately 1 cm proximal to the tip.

Blood pressure (arterial)
The pressure of the blood as it pulsates through the arteries.

Body surface area (BSA)
One of the indices used in the calculation of cardiac output.

Bradycardia
An abnormally slow heart rate, usually less than 60 bpm.

Bundle of His
Part of the heart's conduction system. It is located between the atrioventricular node and the bifurcation of the right and left bundle branches.

Cardiac index
A guide used to evaluate an individual's cardiac output. It is obtained by dividing cardiac output by body surface area. The normal cardiac index is 2.5–4 L/min per m^2.

Cardiac monitor
An instrument used to display the pattern of the patient's heart beat.

Cardiac output
The volume (litres) of blood pumped into the aorta by the left ventricle each minute.

Cardiogenic shock
Severe failure of the left ventricle following myocardial infarction or ischaemia, or from an abnormality in the heart valves or the cardiac muscle.

Cardiopulmonary resuscitation (CPR)
The cessation of a cardiac arrest situation by initiating basic life support and advanced life support as necessary.

Cardioversion
The delivery of a synchronised electrical shock to the patient's myocardium. Cardioversion is used in the treatment of ventricular arrhythmias.

Chordae tendineae
Fibrous bands of tissue embedded in the papillary muscles and attached to the edge of the valve's leaves in the heart.

Compensatory pause
Associated with a premature ventricular complex firing before the next sinus node emission. There is a delay following the abnormal beat, allowing time for the sinus node to resume its role as the chief pacemaker.

Compliance
Related to the extent that the ventricle is able to distend.

Conductivity
The ability of a cell to transmit an impulse.

Contractility
The ability of the muscle to shorten when stimulated.

Coronary heart disease
Occurs due to partial or complete blockage of one or all of the major coronary arteries supplying the myocardium.

Creatnine kinase (CK)
An enzyme which is emitted from damaged striated muscle. Creatnine kinase has three isoenzymes, one (MB) of which can be measured to ascertain whether or not the patient has suffered a myocardial infarction.

Defibrillation
An unsynchronised electrical shock to the myocardium performed during cardiac emergencies with ventricular arrhythmias, such as ventricular fibrillation and ventricular tachycardia.

Delta wave
The characteristic wave pattern seen in Wolff-Parkinson-White Syndrome. There is a shortened PR interval and a slurring of the base of the R wave.

Demand pacing
A mode of the artifical pacemaker. An impulse from the pacemaker is initiated only when a pre-set RR interval has elapsed without any spontaneous electrical activity from the ventricle.

Depolarisation
A state where the membrane potential is less negative than the resting membrane potential. Ionic movement into the cell precedes contraction.

Diastole
The period when the ventricles of the heart are relaxed.

Diffusion
The movement of gases or other particles from areas of greater pressure or concentration to areas of lesser pressure or concentration.

Dyspnoea
Difficulty in breathing. Patients tend to complain that they are short of breath.

Ectopic
An abnormal site; in the case of an ectopic beat, it is initiated from a site outside of the normal conduction pathway. The term *premature ventricular contraction* is synonymous with *ventricular ectopic beat.*

Einthoven's law
This law states that if the electrical potentials of any two of the three bipolar limb leads are known at any given time, by using mathematics and noting the polarity of the leads, the third bipolar limb lead can be determined by adding the first two.

Einthoven's triangle
A triangle drawn around the heart. It is a way of demonstrating that the left arm, the right arm and the left leg form apexes of a triangle surrounding the heart.

Electrocardiogram (ECG)
A graphic recording of the heart's electrical activity.

Electrocardiography
The study of the heart's electrical patterns.

Electrode
An object placed on the skin surface which is capable of sensing a positive wave of electrical movement.

Electrophysiological study
An invasive procedure used to detect abnormal conduction pathways or to evaluate the effectiveness of medication therapy on abnormal rhythms.

Endocardium
The inner lining of the heart.

Epicardium
Covers the external surface of the heart and forms the parietal pericardium.

Excitability
The ability of a cell to respond to an impulse.

Exercise electrocardiography (ECG)
(Also known as a stress test.) Ascertains whether or not the patient has coronary heart disease. Patients are attached to a cardiac monitor and use a treadmill or a stationary bike for the procedure.

Fibrillation
Characterised on the rhythm strip as a chaotic, wavy baseline. The heart chamber with the problem is unable to contract effectively. The condition is caused by multiple ectopic foci firing simultaneously. Ventricular fibrillation is a life-threatening situation and is terminated by emergency defibrillation.

Fixed rate pacing
A type of pacing mode whereby the heart is stimulated at a preset interval. This was the initial method used with artificial pacemakers, but is no longer practised.

Flow
The volume of blood passing a point per unit of time. It is commonly associated with measurement of cardiac output.

Flutter
A type of cardiac rhythm characterised by saw-toothed shaped waves. There are two types of flutter — atrial and ventricular. Atrial flutter originates from a single ectopic focus arising in the walls of the atria which discharges at a rate of 250–400 bpm. The AV node is unable to accept all these impulses and blocks at every second, third or fourth impulse which bombards it. The blocks can be regular — at other times they can be variable. Ventricular flutter is similar to ventricular tachycardia and is life-threatening.

Frank-Starling law
The principle that states that the heart will only pump as much as it is given.

Heart rate
The number of impulses emitted per minute.

Hyperkalaemia
An increased level of potassium in the serum.

Hypertension
Elevated blood pressure where the diastolic pressure exceeds 90 mm/Hg. This condition is a precipitating factor in coronary artery disease.

Hypertrophy
Enlargement of a chamber (eg atrial hypertrophy).

Hypokalaemia
An abnormally low level of serum potassium.

Hypotension
Abnormally low pressure of the blood.

Hypoxia
A reduced level of oxygen in the blood or the tissues.

Ischaemia
Lack of oxygen or blood to the body's tissues.

Isoelectric line
The straight line trace on an ECG trace which includes part of the PR interval and the ST segment. The isoelectric line represents complete muscle depolarisation.

J point
Where the S wave meets the isoelectric line.

Joule
A measurement of the electrical current output.

Lactic dehydrogenase
An enzyme used to ascertain if a patient has had a myocardial infarction.

Lead
The ECG obtained as a result of recording the difference in potential between a pair of electrodes.

Mitral valve
(Also called the *bicuspid valve.*) It is situated between the left atrium and the left ventricle.

Morbidity
The proportion of sickness in the community.

Mortality
The death rate in the community.

Myocardial infarction (MI)
The death of myocardial tissue from lack of oxygen to the tissue as a result of coronary heart disease.

Myocardium
The muscle layer in the heart.

Nomogram
A series of scales arranged so that calculations can be performed graphically.

Nursing diagnosis
An identified patient problem requiring nursing intervention.

P wave
The part of the cardiac cycle which represents atrial depolarisation.

Pacemaker
Either natural or artificial, a pacemaker emits an impulse at a set range per minute. The heart's natural pacemaker is the sinoatrial node. An artificial pacemaker may be inserted to supplement the natural pacemaker, or to act as the heart's pacemaker when the natural one has failed.

Pacing threshold
The lowest level of electrical energy that is required to initiate consistent ventricular capture at the pacing electrode site.

Palpation
The act of feeling with the hands, usually with the tips of the fingers.

Papillary muscle
Muscle bundles embedded in the walls of the ventricles. When they contract, the chordae tendineae are pulled taut.

Parasympathetic nervous system
The part of the autonomic nervous system that tends to increase secretions and dilate blood vessels. It also causes slowing of the heart rate.

Paroxysmal
Occurs abruptly and ends in the same way (eg paroxysmal atrial tachycardia). It may be short-acting or may continue for several hours.

Pericarditis
Inflammation of the pericardium. A normal complication of myocardial infarctions, characterised on the ECG by persistent ST segment elevation. When the patient's chest is auscultated, a sound similar to rubbing together strands of hair can be heard — a scratchy type of noise. Patients often experience chest pain, but unlike the pain of infarction, it is relieved by mild analgesia and change of position.

Pericardium
Part of the outer surface of the heart. It is also attached to the sternum and the ligaments of the diaphragm. The pericardium maintains the position of the heart within the chest cavity and helps to prevent the spread of disease to the heart from other areas of the body.

Practitioner
Related to a medical practitioner (doctor) or a nurse practitioner. The nurse should have at least 10 years experience and be considered by their peers, including the registering authority, as an expert in their field. The practitioner should possess appropriate qualifications as deemed necessary by the registering authority. The term practitioner is often used freely and is applied to all those who care for people in the health care sector.

Precordial
Pertains to the chest wall, particularly in relation to the precordial chest leads in an ECG.

Preload
The degree of stretch in the myocardial fibres at the end of the phase of diastole.

PR interval
The measure from the beginning of the P wave up to the beginning of the R wave. If there is a Q wave present, the interval is measured from the beginning of the P wave up to the beginning of the Q wave. The interval represents the time it takes for the impulse to leave the sinoatrial node and to spread through the atria to the atrioventricular node. This normally takes 0.12–0.20 seconds.

Pulmonary valve
Located between the right ventricle and the pulmonary artery.

Purkinje fibres
The terminal part of the heart's conduction system.

QRS complex
Represents ventricular depolarisation.

QT interval
Part of the cardiac cycle. The QT interval is measured from the beginning of the Q wave to the end of the T wave. It should measure less than 0.42 seconds if the heart rate is 60–95 bpm. If the heart rate is faster, then a nomogram should be used to rate the correct QT interval.

Refractoriness
A term applied to the heart's ability to maintain a steady rhythm by blocking the effects of a stronger than normal electrical stimulus which would initiate a further contraction by the heart.

Registered nurse (RN)
One who holds the necessary qualifications of a recognised hospital certificate, a diploma or a Bachelor's degree in Nursing and who has satisfied the requirements of the registering authority. The full title is State Registered Nurse (SRN).

Relative refractory period
A term applied when the heart is in the final stages of repolarisation and is able to respond to a stronger than normal stimulus, such as a ventricular ectopic beat.

Repolarisation
The return of the cell's membrane to its resting potential.

Resting membrane potential
The period at the end of repolarisation when the membrane is relatively permeable to sodium ions.

Rhythm
A beat occurring at regular intervals.

ST segment
The part of the isoelectric line between the end of the S wave and the beginning of the T wave.

Signal averaged ECG (SAECG)
A special type of ECG which is able to detect repolarisation delays in patients susceptible to ventricular arrhythmias following a myocardial infarction.

Sinoatrial (SA) node
The pacemaker of the heart, normally discharging an impulse at the rate of 60–100 bpm when the patient is at rest.

Standardisation of the electrocardiogram
Before a recording of the heart's electrical activity is performed, the ECG is normally standardised to 1 mV or 10 mm deflection of the trace by pressing the appropriate button on the ECG machine. Without this mark, the ECG cannot be interpreted correctly.

Stenosis
The narrowing of a vessel or a heart valve.

Stroke volume
The volume of blood pumped with each heart beat.

Sympathetic nervous system
Part of the autonomic nervous system that tends to decrease secretions and affects the heart by increasing the rate and the force of contraction.

Synchronised
The delivery of an electrical countershock during the QRS complex in order to prevent competition and the initiation of life-threatening arrhythmias if the shock is delivered on the peak of the T wave.

Synchronous pacing
This occurs when one chamber of the heart is stimulated to fire or is inhibited by the other chamber's activity.

Syncope
A temporary loss of consciousness usually due to decreased cardiac output.

Systole
The period when the ventricles of the heart are contracting.

Tachycardia
A resting heart rate of 100–180 bpm (eg sinus tachycardia). However, tachycardias can be defined as any resting heart rate above 100 bpm.

Thallium isotope
A radionuclide. Thallium-201 is injected into the patient's vein during an exercise test to see how well the coronary arteries allow blood to perfuse the heart. A few minutes are allowed to elapse and the patient is then taken to a special room where the patient's arteries are scanned. The amount of thallium-201 which is injected is not enough to make the patient radioactive and patients should be reassured of this.

Tricuspid valve
The valve between the right atrium and the right ventricle.

Trigeminy
Two normal consecutive sinus node beats followed by a ventricular ectopic beat.

T wave
Part of the ECG complex. The T wave is the rounded upward deflection following the ST segment and represents ventricular repolarisation.

Unipolar catheter
Compared to the bipolar catheter, this variety of catheter only has a negative pacing electrode at its tip. The positive pole is outside the catheter itself. Most permanent pacemakers use a unipolar catheter and the generator box is the positive pole.

U wave
A small upright wave that follows the T wave and when present may be indicative of hypokalaemia.

Vasoconstriction
A decrease in the lumen of the blood vessels.

Vasodilation
An increase in the lumen of the blood vessels.

Ventricle
The lower chamber of the heart. There are two ventricles, one on each side of the septum. The right ventricle ejects deoxygenated blood into the pulmonary artery via the pulmonary valve and the left ventricle ejects oxygenated blood into the aorta via the aortic valve.

Wolff-Parkinson-White Syndrome
A congenital arrhythmia, characterised by a rapid heart rate. Wolff-Parkinson-White Syndrome is due to an accessory electrical pathway, the bundle of Kent, which is located either in the right atrial wall extending into the top of the right ventricle (type A) or in the left atrial wall extending into the top of the left ventricle (type B). When stimulated, the bundle of Kent intercepts the impulse from the sinoatrial node and takes it via this electrical pathway (which is a quicker route) to the ventricles.

INDEX

A
Absolute refractory period 193
Action potential 193
Action potential curve 67
Acute myocardial infarction 133, 193
  aetiology 135
  anterior
    septal 144
    electrocardiogram (ECG) 17, 141–4
    electrocardiographic diagnosis 137
    enzyme levels 136
    infarction 133, 139, 142
    inferior infarction 138, 140–3
    lateral infarction 135–40
    pericarditis 27, 199
    posterior 140
    site of 135–40
    stages of infarction 133, 137
    transmural infarction (Q wave infarction) 133, 138
Advanced life support (ALS) 193
Afterload 11–12, 193
Ambulatory ECG 43–4
  Holter monitor 43–4
Ambulatory monitoring 193
Amiodarone 108
  effects on ECG complex 26
Aneurysm 193
Antiarrhythmic medications 108–10, 193
  classifications 108
Aorta 3–4, 8, 11
  aortic valve 3–4, 193
Arrhythmias 58–94, 115–29, 193
  accelerated idioventricular rhythm 82–3
  accelerated junctional rhythm 73–4
  atrial ectopic beat 67–8
  atrial fibrillation 70–1
  atrial flutter 69–70
    bundle branch block 90–3
    cardiac rhythm answers 172–3, 174–86
    cardiac rhythm exercises 150–65
    cardiac rhythm interpretation 95
    emotional response 114
  first degree AV block 84–6
  junctional ectopic beat 72–3
  junctional tachycardia 74–5
  paroxysmal atrial tachycardia 74–5
  SA arrest or block 64–5
  second degree AV block (type II) 87
  second degree AV block (Wenckebach) 86
  sinus arrhythmia 63
  sinus bradycardia 60–1
  sinus rhythm 29–30, 58–9
  sinus tachycardia 62
  third degree AV block 88–9
  ventricular asystole 81
  ventricular bigeminy 78
  ventricular ectopic beat 76–8
  ventricular fibrillation 80–1
  ventricular standstill 81
  ventricular tachycardia 78–9
  Wolff-Parkinson-White Syndrome 52–3
Arteriole 194
Aspartate transaminase 194
  see also cardiac enzyme
Asynchronous 66–8, 123, 194
Atherosclerosis 194
Atria 2
Atrial ectopic beat 67–8
Atrial fibrillation 70–1
Atrial flutter 69–70
Atrioventricular (AV) node 194
Atrioventricular universal pacing 124, 194
Atrium 2–4, 194
Atropine sulphate 61, 87, 88
Auscultation 194
Automatic implantable cardioverter/defibrillator (AICD) 117–20
Automaticity 194

B
Bainbridge reflex 194
Basic life support (BLS) 194
Beta blocker 71, 108
Biphasic wave 21–2

Bifocal pacing 124, 194
Bigeminy 194
Bipolar catheter 194
Blood pressure 194
Body surface area (BSA) 194
Bradycardia 195
Bundle of His 195

C
Cardiac arrest 80–2, 111–12, 117
Cardiac cycle 10
Cardiac enzyme 136
Cardiac index 195
Cardiac monitoring 44, 195
  alarm system 48
  basic cardiac monitor 44–6
    components of 45–6
    electrical interference 46
    electrical precautions 127
    electrodes 42, 43, 46–8
    false alarms 46
    Holter monitor 43
    monitoring leads 46–8
    operation of monitors 44–6
    telemetry 42–3
Cardiac output 11, 120, 195
Cardiac pacing 120
  loss of 128–9
  rate of 121
  see also transvenous
Cardiogenic shock 195
Cardiopulmonary resuscitation (CPR) 195
Cardioversion 117
  energy of discharge 117, 195
  equipment required 115
    indications for use 117
    sedation and anaesthesia 117
    technique 115–16
Chest pain 133, 135
Chordae tendineae 195
Circumflex artery 5
Compensatory pause 195
Compliance 12, 195
Conductivity 195
Contractility 9, 195
Coronary artery 5, 135
Coronary blood flow 5–6
Coronary care unit (CCU) 42
  cardiac monitoring 44, 108, 110, 113, 127
  defibrillator 115
Coronary heart disease 135, 195
  acute myocardial infarction 135
  creatnine kinase (CK and CKMB) 136, 195
  aetiology 135

D
Defibrillation 115, 195
  automatic implantable cardioverter/ defibrillator (AICD) 117–20
  equipment required 115
  technique 115
  ventricular fibrillation 80–3, 112, 115
  ventricular tachycardia 80–3, 112, 115
Delta wave 196
Diastole 196
Diffusion 196
Digitalis toxicity 18, 27, 108
Diphasic 26
Disorders of conduction 84
Dyspnoea 101, 196

E
Einthoven's law 196
Einthoven's triangle 19
Electrical safety *see* microshock
Electrocardiography (ECG) 14–39, 196
  12 lead electrocardiogram (ECG) 7–24, 136, 140–4, 193
  arrhythmias 108
  basic principles of 15
  configuration of normal ECG complex 24
  diagnosis of acute myocardial infarction 137
  diagnosis of acute myocardial injury 138
  disturbances of conduction 31, 84
  disturbances of impulse formation 30
  ECG leads 18
  electrocardiogram (ECG) 17
  exercise test (stress test) 49–52
  interpretation of cardiac arrhythmias 29
  monitoring leads 46
  signal averaged ECG (SAECG) 140
  site of myocardial infarction 139
  wave forms 20–8
Electrodes 196
  for cardiac monitoring 46
  catheter for electrophysiological studies 54
Electrophysiological studies 52–5, 196
Endocardium 2, 4, 196
Epicardium 2, 4, 196
Excitability 197
Exercise testing 49–52, 197

F
Fibrillatory waves *see* atrial fibrillation
Fibrillation 197
First degree AV block 84–6
Fixed rate pacing 197
Flow 197
Flutter 197
Flutter waves *see* atrial flutter
Frank-Starling law 197

G
Glyceral trinitrate 114

H
Heart block 84
  atrioventricular (AV) 84
  in the sinoatrial (SA) node 64, 65
  see also disorders of conduction
Heart rate 197
Heart sounds 104, 105
  murmurs 104
  normal sounds 105
Holter monitor 43–4
Hyperkalaemia 27, 108, 197
Hypertension 197
Hypertrophy 197
Hypokalaemia 27, 79, 80, 197
Hypotension 197
Hypoxia 197

I
Idioventricular rhythm 82
  accelerated 83
Infarction 33, 138
  anterior 138–42
  anterior lateral (anterolateral) 140, 144
  anterior septal (anteroseptal) 140
  inferior 138, 140–3
  lateral 138, 140
  posterior 140
  reduction of size 114
  right ventricle 2–4
  septal 140
  subendocardial (non Q wave) 138, 141
  transmural (Q wave) 138
Ischaemia 17, 26–7, 138, 139, 141, 197
Isoelectric line 198
Isoprenaline 86

J
J point 24–5, 198
Joule 198
Jugular venous pressure 106–7
Junctional arrhythmia 71–5
Junctional ectopic beat 72–3

L
Lactic dehydrogenase 136, 198
Lead 198
Left anterior descending coronary artery 5
Left main coronary artery 5
Left ventricular failure 60–70
Left ventricular hypertrophy 18, 27
Lignocaine 108
  in treatment of ventricular ectopic beats 77
  ventricular tachycardia 80

M
Magnesium sulphate 77, 80
Microshock 127
Mitral valve 198
Mobitz type II heart block 87
Monitoring equipment 44
Morbidity 198
Morphine 133
Mortality 198
  coronary heart disease 135
Myocardial infarction (MI) 198
Myocardial injury 138–41
Myocardial ischaemia 27, 138–41, 197
  electrocardiographic signs 127, 139
  stress testing 51
Myocardium 198

N
Nomogram 198
Nursing care
  during monitoring procedures 42–55
  emotional support 114
  in cardiac pacing 109–14, 127–9
  in elective cardioversion 116
  in emergency defibrillation 109–15
  in patients experiencing arrhythmias 109–14
Nursing diagnosis 198

P
Pacemaker 198
Pacing 120–9
  atrioventricular (AV) 124, 125
  codes 124–5
  complications 128–9
  demand 196
  electrical safety 128
  equipment required 121, 127
  indications for 120
  modes 123–4
  pacing wire 121
  permanent 121–3, 127–8
  temporary 127–8
  transcutaneous 123
  threshold 198
  transvenous 123, 127–8
Palpation 198
Papillary muscle 198
Parasympathetic nervous system 199
Paroxysmal 199
Paroxysmal atrial tachycardia 68, 69
Paroxysmal junctional tachycardia 74, 75, 199
Pathological Q wave 26, 137, 138
Pericardial space 4
Pericarditis 27, 199
Pericardium 2, 4, 199
Practitioner 199
Precordial 199
Preload 12
PR interval 199
Propranolol 71, 108
Pulmonary valve 199
Purkinje fibres 199
Pulse deficit 106
Pulse pressure 106

Q
QRS complex 199
QT interval 199
Quinidine 17
effect on ECG complex 108

R
Relative refractory period 200
Respiratory assessment 103
Resting membrane potential 200
Resuscitation
cardiopulmonary 80–2, 111–12
during electrophysiological studies 53–5
during stress testing 51
emergency defibrillation; staff responsibilities 51–5
R on T phenomena *see* ventricular ectopic beat

S
Second degree AV block (Mobitz type II) 87
Second degree AV block (Wenckebach) 86
Signal averaged ECG (SAECG) 140, 200
Sinoatrial (SA) node block 64, 65
Sinus arrhythmia 63
Sinus bradycardia 60, 61
Sinus tachycardia 62
Sotalol 77, 108
ST depression 27, 138
ST elevation 27, 137–8
Stenosis 200
Streptokinase 134
Stress testing *see* exercise testing
ST segment 200
Sympathetic nervous system 200
Syncope 200
Systole 201
Synchronisation *see* cardioversion
Synchronous pacing 123

T
Tachycardia 201
Telemetry 42–3
Thallium-201 radioisotope 51–2, 201
Third degree AV block 88–9
Thrombus 135
Tissue plasminogen activator 134
Torsades de Pointes *see* ventricular tachycardia
Transcutaneous 123
Transvenous 123–8
Tricuspid valve 201
Tridil (glyceryl trinitrate) 134
Trigeminy 201
T wave inversion 25, 27, 137, 139, 201

U
Unipolar catheter 201
U waves 28
significance of 28

V
Valves 2–4
aortic 2–4, 193
mitral 2–4, 198
pulmonary 2–4, 199
tricuspid 2–4, 201
Vasoconstriction 201
Vasodilation 201
Ventricle 201
Ventricular ectopic beat 76–8
Ventricular fibrillation 80–1
automatic implantable cardioverter/defibrillator (AICD) 117–20
emergency defibrillation 80–1, 109–15, 129
Ventricular rupture 55
Ventricular standstill 81
Ventricular tachycardia 78–9
Verapramil 70

W
Wandering pacemaker 65–6
Wolff-Parkinson-White Syndrome 52–3, 201